Essential Kidney Diet Skills Every Dialyzor Needs To Know

The Beginners' Guide
For How To Eat A Low Potassium, Low Phosphorus,
And/or Low Sodium Diet

Susan & William Emeny

Susan & William Emeny

Kidney Diet Skills Every Dialyzor Needs To Know
First Edition 2021

SAGE Publishing

Paperback ISBN: 978-0-9886815-0-7
e-Book ISBN: 978-0-9886815-2-1

DEDICATION

To my hero and the love of my life, my husband Bill.

If it wasn't for him, I might not be here today. Bill, Thank you from the bottom of my heart.

Susan & William Emeny

Contents

DEDICATION iii

Introduction: What The Heck Can I Eat? 10

Chapter 1: So, Why A Kidney Diet? 12

   The Benefits of Following A Kidney Diet 15

Chapter 2: So, What Is A Kidney Diet? 17

   Diet Guidelines:...18

Chapter 3: How to Follow A Kidney Diet......................................21

   Kidney Diet Control 21

   What you need to do: 21

   Daily Limits 21

   Weight of food items: 23

   Where to buy a scale: 23

   Nutrient values of protein, phosphorous, potassium and sodium
   for each food item. 23

   The hard way:..23

   The Easy Way 28

   Recording Daily Nutrient Values 30

   Breakfast and Lunch Nutrition Chart 31

   Recording Total Daily Nutrient Values 32

Chapter 4: The Kidney Diet Explained..34

   Big Mac: 35

   Small French fry: 36

   Big Mac meal:...36

Breakfast Nutrition:..37

Breakfast and Lunch Nutrition: 37

Chapter 5: Food, Processed Foods and Shopping 39

What should I eat? 39

Deli Roast Beef Nutrition: 40

What You Need To Do:...40

Meat Nutrition Values:..42

Vegetable Nutrition Values: 42

Starchy Food Nutrition Values: 42

Drinks Nutrition Values:......................................42

Condiment Nutrition Values: 43

Breakfast Example: 43

Lunch Example: 45

Supper Example: 46

Atkins Cookies n' Crème Bar 48

Pork Pot Roast Recipe: 49

Pork Pot Roast Nutrients:...................................49

Pork Pot Roast Gravy Recipe:.............................49

Pork Pot Roast Gravy Nutrients: 49

Processed Foods and Shopping...........................50

Kidney Bean Nutrition:.......................................52

Home Cooking:...55

Homemade White Bread vs Store Bought White Bread. 55

Chili Powder Comparison:...................................56

Eating Out: 56

Fish Fry Dinner Nutrition: 56

Steak Dinner Nutrition: 58

Pork Chop Dinner Nutrition: 58

Chapter 6: Recipes 60

Beef and Peppers 61

Beef Stew 62

Beef and Vegetables 63

Beef, Roast 64

Beef, Roast Beef Sandwich, Deli Beef 65

Beef, Roast Beef Sandwich, homemade beef 66

Beef, Teriyaki Beef and Peppers 67

Bread, White Homemade Bread 68

Chicken Stir Fry with General Toas Sauce 69

Corn Bread 70

Fish, Baked Haddock 71

Hamburg and Gravy 72

Hamburg and Gravy with Vegetables 73

Macaroni and Cheese 74

Meatballs, Italian 75

Meatloaf..76

Meatloaf Sauce 77

Omelet with Pepperoni...78

Pork Pot Roast..79

Pork Pot Roast Gravy 80

Pork, General Toas 81

Pork, General Toas Stir Fry.......................................82

General Toas Sauce 83

Red Cabbage, Prepared..84

Fried Rice...85

Rubin Sandwich with Red Cabbage............................86

Salsa, Homemade from Cans 87

Sauce, Spaghetti Sauce with Meat.............................88

Sausage, Breakfast Homemade, Low Salt 89

Sausage, Breakfast Sausage Seasoning, Low Salt........90

Sausage, Hot Italian Homemade 91

Sausage Seasoning, Hot Italian 92

Scrapple 93

Soup, Lentil 94

Taco Meat 95

Teriyaki Sauce 96

Tuna and Noodles 97

Tuna, Creamed...98

Chapter 7: Resources to Get More Info 99

Chapter 8: Weight & Measures Equivalent Chart 100

Chapter 9: Nutrient List...101

About the Authors 102

Bill 102

Susan 102

Introduction: What The Heck Can I Eat?

If you are struggling with a kidney diet, then you need to read this book. Not knowing what to do is scary. Take the time to read through the following pages and start learning what to do and how to cope.

I will give you a lot of the information you need to know. I will show you where to find the nutrition information you need, and I will show you how to use it. It is not as hard as you may think. So, to reduce your stress level, read on.

Hi. I'm Sue Emeny and you are probably wondering how I am qualified to be offering my help. The short story is that I spent eight years at the school of hard knocks. I learned how to cope with dialysis and how to eat properly. Just like you, I was not given much information about diet. I was just told to watch what I ate. There was no mention of how to do it.

Let me tell you a little bit about myself. Before I had to start dialysis, I was working as a software engineer and my dream was to tour the country with my horse. Then the bottom fell out from under me. I was getting weaker and more tired by the day. I didn't know why. Then I was told I had to start dialysis soon and start the process for a kidney transplant. I had to quit work and I could no longer ride my horse.

I started dialysis on July 26, 2012 and remained on dialysis until September 22, 2019 when I got a kidney transplant. During the time before I had to dialyze, I learned a lot about following a kidney diet. I learned enough that I put dialysis off for about four months. How did I do that?

Well, I am a career software engineer with over thirty years' experience writing programs for just about anything you can think of. My husband is also an engineer, so we got our heads together and decided to learn how to do a kidney diet.

We were successful. We discovered the secret of eating with kidney failure. I wrote a software App to get nutrition information from the USDA food database. I wrote an App to keep track of everything I ate during the day. I wrote another App to evaluate all our recipes.

My husband and caregiver evaluated all our recipes and revised many of them to reduce sodium. We paid close attention to what I ate all the time I was on dialysis. The result was that my life on dialysis was made much easier.

I am not a dietitian, but I have gained a lot of knowledge about eating when you have kidney disease. I would very much like to pass that knowledge on to you. In fact my goal in writing this book is to help other people discover how to eat well with kidney failure.

There are many benefits to learning about diet. The most important one is that you will feel better. You also will stop worrying about what you can eat, because you will know. You will be able to eat the foods that you like and are used to. Diet knowledge when you are on dialysis is the key to a better life.

Chapter 1: So, Why A Kidney Diet?

Quality of life is a big issue when you are dealing with kidney failure and dialysis. There is a direct relationship between diet, treatment, quality of life and your overall well-being.

It is really important that you or anybody facing or experiencing dialysis understands the connection between their diet, their lab results, their dialysis prescription and how they feel after treatment. By doing so, you are more likely to experience a better quality of life and be able to eat a larger variety of foods and/ or bigger portions.

Since the kidneys no longer function properly, or at all, dialysis is used to remove toxins and to maintain proper levels of fluid, potassium, phosphorous and sodium (salt). Dialysis is not easy on your body. The more dialysis needed to maintain proper levels of fluid, potassium, phosphorous and sodium the lousier you are likely to feel.

While on dialysis you will have a prescription that defines how much fluid and other nutrients are going to be removed from your blood. The more you eat over your dietary limits the more that has to be removed. This makes the treatment harsher which in turn makes you feel worse when it is done. The more fluid that has to be removed means that you will have to dialyze longer or remove liquid faster. The faster you remove fluid the worse you are going to feel.

Getting the right prescription takes time and cooperation with your doctor and dietitian. You will most likely initially be given a prescription based on your weight, gender, and body mass. You will be expected to follow the dietary guidelines which they may or may not give you. You need to insist that they give them to you. The prescription is not easily changed.

Your labs are normally reviewed only once a month which makes it important that you consistently stay within your dietary limits. If you don't, you will feel lousy and put your well-being in jeopardy. Diet affects your prescription requirements because a good diet results in good lab results. Eating habits are in your control, but your dialysis prescription is up to your doctor. If you have consistently good labs, you are more likely to gain his trust and he is more likely to adjust your prescription to make dialysis easier on you. I know this from personal experience.

A proper diet makes a huge difference. Take it from someone who has suffered through dialysis and has benefited from eating correctly.

Let's talk about fluids and potassium, phosphorous and sodium.

Fluids. Your body needs fluids but not too much. What your body doesn't use normally ends up as urine. But now with kidney failure, you can't pee enough or not at all, so you have to depend on dialysis to remove it. It is way better not to drink excess fluid than it is to dialyze it off.

When there is too much fluid in your body it is very easy to fall into the trap of taking off too much fluid too fast. The result is hypotension (low blood pressure) and you can pass out because of it. It has happened to me a couple of times and it is really scary. When this happens, you will probably be given fluid to fix it. This results in not getting enough fluid off. Removing excess fluid is stressful on the body and makes you feel lousy.

The more water in your body the more likely you are to bloat which can cause high blood pressure. You are always fighting blood pressure on dialysis. In fact, rising blood pressure often means you are retaining fluid.

So, don't drink too much fluid. Water, coffee, tea, soda is on the restricted list. All the while I was on dialysis, I limited myself to drinking no more than one liter of fluid a day.

Too much Sodium (salt) causes water retention and bloating. It also makes you thirsty and makes you want to drink more. Too much sodium in your diet may cause cramping, especially for patients on in-center hemodialysis. This can be very painful, and you will probably be given fluid to stop the cramping and again you are likely to end up with too much fluid at the end of your treatment. So be smart and limit the salt in your diet.

Potassium needs close attention. Too much is bad and so is too little. High potassium can cause irregular heartbeat, potential heart attack and/or diarrhea. Low potassium can cause weak muscles, nausea, heart problems, and even high blood pressure. Low potassium made me feel really lousy, especially right after treatment.

Phosphorus if too high, can cause calcified organs, weakened bones, bone pain, itching, and muscle weakness. Too little phosphorus can cause appetite loss and confusion.

Protein is another nutrient that you need to watch. Too little protein can cause weakness, muscle loss and a weakened immune system. Your protein requirements will change depending on which type of dialysis you are doing. Insist that your doctor or dietitian tells you how much protein you should be eating every day.

Adjusting to failed kidneys is no picnic and it will certainly alter your way of life. There is a lot to learn and there are a lot of old habits to adjust. You can maintain a good quality of life if you learn to control the blood levels of protein, potassium (K+), phosphorus (Phos), and sodium (Na).

One of the traps many dialyzors fall into is overeating on holidays and family or friend get-togethers. The first treatment in a dialysis center after an overindulgence, is seldom a good one.

What you eat or don't eat and how much you eat or don't eat is hugely important and directly affects your quality of life.

The Benefits of Following A Kidney Diet

There is a direct relationship between diet and quality of life. The more attention you pay to your diet the better you are going to feel. The more you understand about diet the easier it will be to make it fit your individual dialysis prescription.

Here are a few of the benefits of following a kidney diet that has been fitted to your dialysis prescription.

1. You will feel better.
2. Your dialysis prescription can be more easily changed to better fit your needs and wellbeing.
3. Dialysis will be easier on your body with less fluid, phosphorous, potassium and sodium to be removed. The less you have to remove, the better you will feel.
4. You will more likely avoid the issues of phosphorous, potassium and sodium being out of their normal range. This is important because it can be life threatening. It also makes you feel lousy.
5. You will be able to eat foods that you like but probably not

as much as you wish you could.

6. You will have peace of mind in knowing that you are helping yourself by doing what's best for you with no more uncertainty about doing it wrong.

Gain the trust and respect of your doctor when you show him/her exactly what you are eating. It helps him/her to do his/her job. It also makes it more likely that he will agree to change your prescription to be less harsh on your body. To do this, he has to know that you are paying attention and have the knowledge to keep yourself safe. I've experienced this firsthand with several different doctors. It has been very worthwhile for me.

Is it worth it to follow a kidney diet? For me, it was a resounding YES!

Chapter 2: So, What Is A Kidney Diet?

A kidney diet is a diet that is paired with your dialysis prescription. It is intended to help you to get a sufficient amount of protein and maintain the proper levels of fluid, phosphorus, potassium, and sodium in your blood.

A kidney diet has two parts. The first part is about choosing the foods that will allow you to stay within your nutritional limits. The second part is about portion control. You can eat small amounts of the bad stuff and more of the good stuff and stay within your nutritional limits.

I will tell you how to stay within your daily limits and eat just about anything you want. I will also tell you not to eat too much of the "bad" stuff in one sitting. The key is portion control, and I will talk about this in detail. I will also teach you how to get nutrient values for protein, phosphorous, potassium and sodium. I will show you how to use this information to stay within your daily limits.

I will use some of my own nutrition data from my diet when I was in Center to show you how to use your nutrition information to improve your well-being.

In addition, I will include a meal plan for one day and use it to illustrate how I still control my kidney diet even though I recently got a transplant.

The technique that I am going to show you works for a diabetic diet as well as a diet to just watch your weight.

I will tell you how to follow a diet in the next chapter. So, read on.

Diet Guidelines:

Your doctor or dietitian will need to recommend specific guidelines for the daily amounts of phosphorus, potassium, sodium, and protein for your diet. You may also have a daily limit of the amount of fluid you can drink. I had to ask for these amounts, they were NOT volunteered.

Talk to your medical team. Get your specific dietary requirements. Insist on it if necessary.

The daily guidelines I badgered out of my doctor were:

- 2000 milligrams of sodium
- 2000 milligrams of potassium
- 1000 milligrams of phosphorus
- 60 grams (g) of protein.
- 1000 grams of water (I added this myself to shorten my dialysis time)

Guidelines may be different for you. They depend on the type of dialysis you are doing, your body size and weight. Again, get your specific guidelines from your doctor or dietitian. The chart below shows the general rules of thumb for dietary guidelines contributed by my dietitian.

	In Center	PD	Home Hemo SDD	HHD Nocturnal
Potassium	2000 mg	Usually No Restriction		No Restriction
Phosphorus	1000mg	1000 mg	1000 mg	May have to eat more!
Protein	1.2 -1.4g*	1.4 - 1.6g*	1.2g*	1.4+ g*
Sodium	2000 mg	2000 mg	2000 mg	2000 mg

General Rules of Thumb for Dietary Limitations   *Per kg of body weight

1. PD is peritoneal dialysis
2. Home Hemo SDD is Home Hemodialysis Short Daily Dialysis

3. HHD Nocturnal is Home Hemodialysis Nocturnal; done at night for a longer period of time and at a slower rate.
4. kg is kilogram and equals 1000 grams and equals 2.2 pounds

Don't let the use of metric weights turn you off. I know that 2000 mg (milligram) of potassium doesn't mean anything to you, but then neither would 1/16 ounce of potassium.

Don't worry about the use of milligrams or grams, just think of it as a number you need to achieve. You will just have to weigh your food on a metric scale which is easily available at Amazon.

Now What? Here comes the hard part. You have to learn to use the tools that are available to track your daily nutrition (diet). I will tell you how in the next chapter.

The USDA Food Data Central is a government-maintained database of food's nutritional values for protein, phosphorus, potassium, sodium, calories, fat, water, carbohydrates, fiber, and sugars. It is available for free to anyone that wants to use it. You can look up the nutritional values of the food you eat, which will help you to keep track of your daily totals of phosphorus, potassium, sodium, and protein. I will give you a link in the next chapter and explain how to use it.

You need to record everything you eat and drink. You can use a spreadsheet, either an electronic one or a piece of paper. This is a slow and tedious process, but it is doable. Again, I will show you how in the next chapter.

There are more and more recipes being published that provide the nutrition information that you need to track your diet.

Be careful when using them. The weight of a serving is not always given. Without it, you will not know how much of a serving you are eating, and you will not have the nutrition values you need to track your diet.

One book I looked at only provided nutrition information for a serving size. It did not tell me what a serving size was. It did tell me how many servings there were to a recipe, but no weight.

So, if I want to know the weight of a serving size, I will have to weigh the entire recipe and then divide by the number of servings. Then I would have to scale each nutrient accordingly.

Now I can eat however much I want and get the nutrition information I need.

It would have to be a really good recipe for me to bother to do that. It would be just about as easy to get the values for one of my own recipes that I know I like.

There is an App available that makes it easy to find food in the USDA database and makes it easy to use. I will talk about that in the next chapter as well.

Chapter 3: How to Follow A Kidney Diet

Kidney Diet Control

It's time to start on this adventure into the wilderness of nutrition. So here is a list of what you have to do. I hope you are ready for a lifestyle change because failed kidneys pretty much forces you to do it.

What you need to do:

1. Know your daily limits for protein, phosphorous, potassium and sodium.
2. Weigh and record everything you eat and drink.
3. Find and record nutrient values of protein, phosphorous, potassium and sodium for each food item you eat.
4. Keep daily totals of the fluids you drink and the nutrient values of protein, phosphorous, potassium and sodium you have eaten.

Don't panic, you can do this. I did it and I didn't have any help or anyone to tell me how to proceed. I am here offering you my help so you don't have to go through what I did.

Daily Limits

For all of the illustrations that I show I will use my personal, prescribed daily limits. I used these daily limits while I was on home hemo dialysis. All of the illustrations that I show are based on these limits. I call them my nutrition budget. Get yours from your doctor or dietitian.

1. Phosphorous   1000 mg (milligrams)
2. Potassium   2000 mg (milligrams)
3. Sodium   2000 mg (milligrams)

4. Protein 60 g (grams)

A word about metric measure: It's easy, don't worry about it, but just in case you do, I will try to explain how it is used in nutrition.

1. 1 gram (gm) is equal to 1000 milligrams (mg)
2. phosphorous, potassium and sodium are always expressed in milligrams (mg)
3. Protein is always expressed in grams (g)
4. The weight of food that you eat is always expressed in grams (g)

Think of phosphorous, potassium and sodium as just a number and the total number that I can eat in a day are my limits or budget. I can eat 1000 Phosphorous.

Protein is the same. It is just a number and I need about 60 of them a day.

Fluid like coffee and water is expressed in grams. I limit myself to 1000 grams of fluid a day which is about 5 cups. Refer to Chapter 8 for more information on weights and measures.

Food items need to be expressed in grams, so be careful to get the gram number from the label. Now it is just a number again. When you weigh food, you will have to use a metric scale. I drink 280 grams of coffee for breakfast and 57 grams of mini wheats with 120g (grams) of milk.

Tip: A good equivalent to remember is that 1ounce equals about 30 grams. (1oz = 30g).

A cup of water weighs 8 ounces or approximately 240 grams. See chapter 8 on weight and measures for more information.

Weight of food items:

To get your nutrition values you are going to have to measure everything on a metric scale. There are good, inexpensive metric kitchen scales available. It is worthwhile to buy one that will weigh in ounces and pounds as well as the metric scales.

Where to buy a scale:

I have used an EatSmart Precision Pro Digital Kitchen Scale for nine years and it works really well for me. They are available at Amazon and Walmart and range in price from $20 to $35.

Nutrient values of protein, phosphorous, potassium and sodium for each food item.

How do I get these values? Let me tell you the ways. There is a hard way and there is an easy way. The hard way is free, and the easy way is not, but the easy way is really worth it. You will understand when you read about both the hard way and the easy way.

The hard way:

You will need a laptop or desktop computer to do this. It is almost impossible to do on a cell phone.

Go to USDA Food Data Central database. Here is the link: https://fdc.nal.usda.gov.

Click on the link or copy-paste it into the address bar of your browser. Press Enter.

See the resulting screen next.

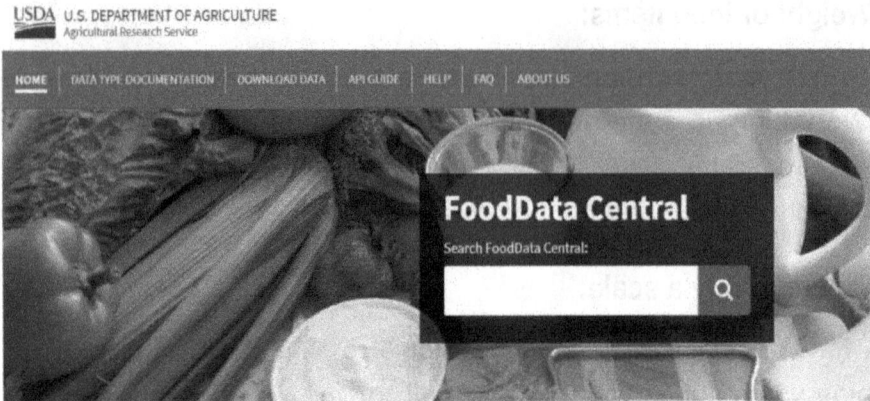

Type pickles in the white box under Food Data Central.

The resulting screen gives you the opportunity to change the search.

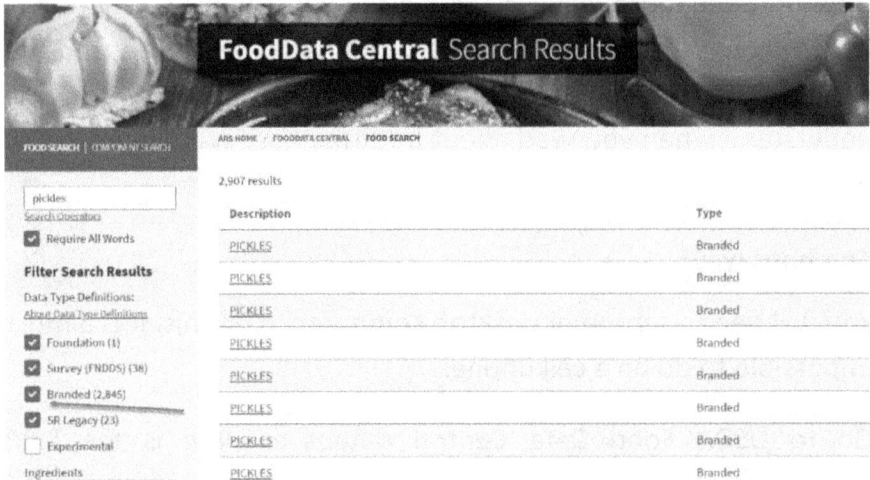

On the left under "Filter Search Results" Click on Branded to turn off these selections.

Branded items are processed foods whose nutrition information is provided by the manufactures, not the USDA. It generally lacks information on phosphorous. An example of Branded food is Campbell's soup.

With "Branded Foods" turned off, the following screen will result and show you a selection of food items to choose from.

1. Scroll down through the list and click on your choice; example "Pickles, Sweet" and view the chart of nutrients in sweet pickle

- ☑ Foundation (1)
- ☑ Survey (FNDDS) (38)
- ☐ Branded (2,865)
- ☑ SR Legacy (23)
- ☐ Experimental

Ingredients

Press enter to search.

Brand Owner

Search Tips

Press enter to search.

Reset   **Search**

Cauliflower, pickled

Celery, pickled

Eggplant, pickled

Eggplant, pickled

Fruit, pickled

Herring, pickled

Mackerel, pickled

Mushrooms, pickled

Okra, pickled

Peppers, pickled

Pickled sausage

Pickles, dill

Pickles, fried

Pickles, sweet

Kidney Diet Skills Every Dialyzor Needs To Know

Portion: | 100g   ⬍ |

Name	Amount	Unit
Water	76.2	g
Energy	91	kcal
Protein	0.58	g
Total lipid (fat)	0.41	g
Carbohydrate, by difference	21.15	g
Fiber, total dietary	1	g
Sugars, total including NLEA	18.27	g
Calcium, Ca	61	mg
Iron, Fe	0.25	mg
Magnesium, Mg	7	mg
Phosphorus, P	18	mg
Potassium, K	100	mg
Sodium, Na	457	mg

2. The portion box shows 100 g meaning 100 grams. The amount column shows how much of each nutrient is in 100 grams of pickle. You will need to scale the amount value if you eat other than 100 grams of pickle.

Be careful and pay attention to the unit column. It lists g for grams and mg for milligrams. Do not mix them up because 1 gram is equal to 1000 milligrams. (1g = 1000mg)

Let me try to explain about scaling; it's not hard. Use the pickle as an example.

Let's calculate the amount of water in 50 grams of pickle.

1. Divide 50 grams of pickle (the amount you are going to eat) by 100 grams (the weight in the chart). This equals 0.5. This is the scale factor for each nutrient.
2. From the chart, the amount of water in 100 grams of pickle is 76.2 grams.
3. Multiply 76.2 gm of water by the scale factor of .5
4. The result is equal to 38.1 grams, which is the amount of water in 50 gm of pickle.
5. Multiply each of the nutrient values that you are tracking, say protein, phosphorous, potassium and sodium by the scale factor .5.
6. Record the results in a spreadsheet, either an electronic one or a paper one.

I found doing this to be time consuming and tedious, so I wrote some software to make it a lot easier.

The Easy Way

The easy way is called KDC Food Finder and it is very easy and quick to use. So, keeping track of your diet is no longer the impossibility it seems.

This is the Food Finder entry page. https://kidneyfoodfinder.com

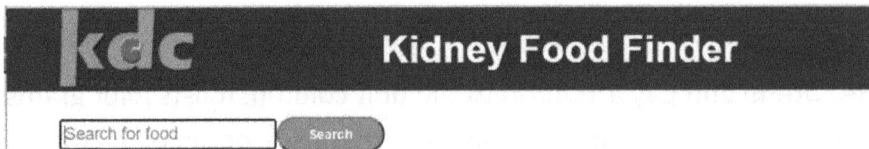

Kidney Diet Skills Every Dialyzor Needs To Know

pickle		Search

Eggplant, pickled	⌄	Choose

Eggplant, pickled
Pickles, cucumber, sweet (includes bread and butter pickles)
Pickle relish, hamburger
Pickle relish, sweet
Pickles, cucumber, sour
Pickles, cucumber, sweet, low sodium (includes bread and butter pickles)
Fish, herring, Atlantic, pickled
Peppers, hot pickled, canned
Pickle and pimiento loaf, pork
Pickle relish, hot dog
Pork, cured, feet, pickled
Pork, pickled pork hocks
Radishes, hawaiian style, pickled
Beets, pickled, canned, solids and liquids
Cabbage, japanese style, fresh, pickled
Olives, pickled, canned or bottled, green
Pickles, cucumber, dill or kosher dill
Pickles, cucumber, dill, reduced sodium
Pickles, cucumber, sour, low sodium
Ginger root, pickled, canned, with artificial sweetener

1. Type Pickles in the white box. Click Search
2. Drop down the choose list
3. Click on Pickles, cucumber, sweet
4. Click on Choose

You get the following chart of pickle nutrients

Grams per Unit of Measure

Qty	Item	Grams
1	large Gherkin (3" long)	35
1	spear Gherkin	20
1	cup, chopped	160
1	cup sliced or chips	153
1	midget Gherkin (2-1/8" long)	6
1	Gherkin (2-3/4" long)	25
1	small Gherkin (2-1/2" long)	15
1	chip	7.5

Enter Serving Size in Grams 75   [Calculate]

Water	Protein	Calories	Fat	Carbs	Fiber	Sugars	Phosphorus	Potassium	Sodium
57.15	0.45	68.25	0.30	15.82	0.75	13.72	13.50	75.00	342.75

Values for Phos., Pot., & Sodium are in mg. All others are in grams

All the information you need to get your nutrition information is there at the bottom of the page.

To get your nutrition information:
1. Weigh the pickles you are eating.
2. Type the weight, into the serving size box
3. Click Calculate The nutrition values are calculated for you.
4. Record the results in a spreadsheet, either an electronic one or a paper one.
5. You are done.

Recording Daily Nutrient Values

To record the nutrient values of each food item you eat you will need a spreadsheet. You can use a paper one or an electronic one like Excel, Google Sheets or Numbers. You will need to record at least:

Food Name, Weight, Fluid, Protein, Phosphorous, Potassium and Sodium

Here is an example spreadsheet of breakfast and lunch. I have used my prescription as an example of Daily Limits.

Breakfast and Lunch Nutrition Chart

											Daily Limits		
	Date:	03/10/19									1000	2000	2000
Qty	Measure	Item	Weight	Water	Calories	Protein	Fat	Carbs	Fiber	Sugars	Phos.*	Pot.*	Sodium*
10	oz	cofee	283.00	282.00	6.00	1.00	0.00	0.00	0.00	0.00	9.00	142.00	3.00
1	tsp	Heavy Cream	5.00	3.00	17.00	0.00	2.00	0.00	0.00	0.00	3.00	5.00	1.00
2	tsp	Sugar	10.00	0.00	39.00	0.00	0.00	10.00	0.00	10.00	0.00	0.00	0.00
1	each	large egg	50.00	38.00	72.00	6.00	5.00	0.00	0.00	0.00	99.00	69.00	71.00
1	each	McDonald's Double Hamburger (calculated)	115.00	48.00	313.00	18.00	17.00	21.00	1.00	575.00	483.00	274.00	483.00
		Daily Totals	463.00	371.00	447.00	25.00	24.00	31.00	1.00	585.00	594.00	490.00	558.00

*Values are in milligrams, all others are in grams

% Daily Totals	59%	25%	28%

*McDonald's hamburger data is not provided by the USDA food data base or McDonalds. It is my calculated estimate based on other data.

Is this a lot of trouble? Yes, it is, but it gets easier. I eat the same breakfast a lot, so I made a breakfast meal called "Breakfast, Egg & Coffee" and used the totals as a line item. Now I only have one line to copy. I use a spreadsheet, so I can just do a copy and paste. I have 3 or 4 breakfasts that I choose from.

I do the same for lunch and supper. I stick to simple easy meals that are quick and easy to prepare. It doesn't take too long to build a library of meals with nutrition values. Once you do, following a diet and tracking your nutrition is pretty easy.

Now that you have your daily nutrition values, you need to use another spreadsheet to track weekly or monthly values. I chose to track from blood draw to blood draw so I could relate nutrition to lab results and how I felt. Tracking how you feel after a meal is very useful when you first start dialysis. I used this information to convince my doctors to pay more attention to me in general and to my prescription in particular.

Recording Total Daily Nutrient Values

You need to record the total daily nutrient values of fluid, protein, phosphorous, potassium and sodium you have eaten. You can use a spreadsheet like the example below. We weren't tracking fat, carbs and sugars back in 2014.

Date	Water	Calories	Protein	Fat	Carbs	Fiber	Sugars	Phos.*	Pot.*	Sodium*
9/21/2014		1506	91					1134	1836	2367
9/22/2014		2039	81					995	2124	3363
9/23/2014	1260	1881	81			4		687	1514	2856
9/24/2020	802	2233	117			2		1302	2398	2115
9/25/2020	750	1894	75			10		1209	1488	3536
9/26/2020	1080	1057	64			24		986	1959	724
Daily Totals	3892	10610	509	0	0	40	0	6313	11319	14961
Daily Average	973	1768	85	0	0	10	0	1052	1887	2494

*Values are in milligrams, all others are in grams

Let's look at the results and see how I am doing.

My water Daily Average of 973 is under my goal of 1000. Protein at 85mg is about right. I was on Peritoneal Dialysis (PD) then with 80 to 90 grams of protein as my goal. Phosphorous at 1052mg is good. Potassium at 1887 mg is below my limit. Sodium at 2494 mg is a big whoops, I had better watch it from now on.

So, you can see the value of keeping track of nutrition. Back in 2014 I was not tracking fat, carbs and sugars, but I decided to extend the tracking to include diabetes menus at a later date.

Why did I go to all this trouble? First of all, I was scared when I was first told that my kidneys were failing and that I needed to watch what I ate. The first few times I tried tracking my diet, I broke my limits really bad and that scared me even more. I found that I felt better when my diet was on track.

Chapter 4: The Kidney Diet Explained

The kidney diet is about what you eat and how much you can eat and not exceed your daily limits or budget.

I like to think of the Kidney Diet as a budget. I have a limit to how much I can eat. If I bust my budget, I pay the consequences. The kidney diet is like counting calories except that you are counting protein, phosphorous, potassium, sodium and fluids.

There is an important issue that the kidney diet does not help with, at least not very much. That is about not eating too much of the "bad" stuff at one time. Bad stuff is phosphorous, potassium and sodium. I should probably include fluid in this list because you pay dearly for drinking too much.

I can't tell you how much of the "bad" stuff is too much because it will be different for just about everybody. Too much bad stuff at a time can make you nauseous and overly tired or sleepy. For example, I cannot eat Greek yogurt without feeling sick.

This is an example of where tracking your diet is important. If you pay attention to how you feel, in particular to when you feel bad, you can see which food is giving you a problem. Now you can avoid it or just eat less at a time. I hope you see where this is leading. If you feel bad, look at your diet and maybe fix it.

The word on the street is that you can't eat foods high in phosphorous, potassium and sodium. This is wrong. The truth is that you can't eat too much of it. This is called portion control and I will talk a lot about it.

Think of the diet as a budget. You only have so much phosphorous, potassium and sodium to spend. If you use most of it on one meal, you will not have much to eat for the rest of the day. This means that you will either be hungry or really bust your diet.

If you decide you have to bust your diet, then make up for it by eating less the day before or the day after or both. If you insist on busting your diet, do it just before dialysis since dialysis will get some of the bad stuff off.

If you do bust your diet, don't do it a day or two before you get you labs drawn. The busted diet will cause a spike in your blood levels and give the doctor a false impression of how well your prescription is working. You do not want him/her changing anything based on wrong information.

I will give you an example of a bad lunch and a good breakfast. For lunch I am going to eat a McDonalds BigMac, a small fry and a small cola. Just so you know, I recommend a double hamburger with no salt instead of a Big Mac, the double hamburger is much better nutrition wise and it only takes McDonalds a couple of extra minutes to cook it.

Here is the nutrition information for a Big Mac right from the USDA Food Data Central database. This is where you get your nutrition data. Here is a link to USDA Food Data Central. https://fdc.nal.usda.gov.

Big Mac:

Enter Serving Size in Grams 269   Calculate

Water	Protein	Calories	Fat	Carbs	Fiber	Sugars	Phosphorus	Potassium	Sodium
136.38	27.44	766.65	52.19	47.07	2.96	2.42	688.64	556.83	1476.81

Values for Phos., Pot., & Sodium are in mg. All others are in grams

Notice the sodium. I have used three quarters of my daily sodium budget.

Here is the nutrition information for a small French fry, also from the USDA Food Data Central database.

Small French fry:

Water	Protein	Calories	Fat	Carbs	Fiber	Sugars	Phosphorus	Potassium	Sodium
25.99	2.41	229.33	11.01	30.25	2.77	0.14	90.17	423.16	134.19

I put the nutrition data for the BigMac, small fries in a spread sheet and the added a cola to make it a BigMac meal with a small soda. Then I added up all the columns.

Big Mac meal:

Qty		Item	Weight	Water	Calories	Protein	Fat	Carbs	Fiber	Sugars	Phos.	Pot.	Sodium
1.00	Each	McDonald's Big Mac	219	112	563	26	33	44	4	9	267	396	1007
1.00	Each	McDonald's French Fry, Small	71	26	229	2	11	30	3	0	90	423	134
12.00	Ounce	Soda, cola, regular	368	329	155	0	1	38	0	37	33	18	11
		Totals	658	468	947	28	45	112	6	45	391	838	1153

Let's look at the data.

1. 2000 sodium (daily limit) minus 1152 sodium leaves 848 for the rest of the day.
2. 2000 potassium (daily limit) minus 838 potassium leaves 1162 for the rest of the day.
3. 1000 phosphorous (daily limit) minus 391 phosphorous leaves 609 for the rest of the day.

If I am striving for an 1800 calorie diet, then I have 854 calories left to eat.

Now I will get my breakfast nutrition.

For breakfast I had coffee with sugar and cream, and a fried egg with toast and butter.

Cream is a better kidney nutrition choice than other choices like half & half.

Breakfast Nutrition:

												Daily Limits		
	Date:											1000	2000	2000
Qty	Measure	Item	Weight	Water	Calories	Protein	Fat	Carbs	Fiber	Sugars	Phos.*	Pot.*	Sodium*
10	oz	cofee	283.00	282.00	6.00	1.00	0.00	0.00	0.00	0.00	9.00	142.00	3.00
1	tsp	Heavy Cream	5.00	3.00	17.00	0.00	2.00	0.00	0.00	0.00	3.00	5.00	1.00
2	tsp	Sugar	10.00	0.00	39.00	0.00	0.00	10.00	0.00	10.00	0.00	0.00	0.00
1	each	large egg	50.00	38.00	72.00	6.00	5.00	0.00	0.00	0.00	99.00	69.00	71.00
1	each	Bread, slice, store	30.00	11.00	80.00	3.00	1.00	15.00	1.00	2.00	29.00	38.00	147.00
1	pat	Butter	5.00	1.00	36.00	0.00	4.00	0.00	0.00	0.00	1.00	1.00	32.00
		Daily Totals	383.00	335.00	250.00	10.00	12.00	25.00	1.00	12.00	141.00	255.00	254.00

*Values are in milligrams, all others are in grams

% Daily Totals	14%	13%	13%

Next, I will add breakfast and lunch together to get my total nutrition so far today.

Breakfast and Lunch Nutrition:

A	B	C	D	E	F	G	H	I	J	K	L
Item	Weight	Water	Calories	Protein	Fat	Carbs	Fiber	Sugars	Phos.*	Pot.*	Sodium*
Sue's Breakfast	383.00	335.00	250.00	10.00	12.00	25.00	1.00	12.00	141.00	255.00	254.00
Lunch; BigMac meal	658.00	467.00	946.00	28.00	45.00	112.00	6.00	46.00	391.00	838.00	1152.00
Daily Totals	1041.00	802.00	1196.00	38.00	57.00	137.00	7.00	58.00	532.00	1093.00	1406.00

*Values are in milligrams, all others are in grams

So how much can we spend for supper?

Item	Used	Limit	Amount Left
1. Water	802	1000	198
2. Calories	1196	1800	604
3. Protein	38	60	22
4. Phosphorous	532	1000	468
5. Potassium	1093	2000	907
6. Sodium	1406	2000	594

So, there we have it. This is an example of how the diet works. I hope I didn't scare you too much with all the charts and numbers. Actually, it is pretty easy once you learn the process and get the tools you need. So please don't give up.

Chapter 5: Food, Processed Foods and Shopping

What should I eat?

The advice I have been given is don't eat processed or pre-packaged food. That pretty much leaves make it from scratch yourself. Not what you wanted to hear, I'm sure. I wasn't very happy with the advice either and it certainly changed my eating habits. Tracking your diet is a pain, finding food to eat is equally difficult or maybe even worse. It is especially difficult if you dialyze in a dialysis center since you will need to follow a stricter diet.

The kidney diet requires portion control. If you are used to eating large meals, you are going to have a difficult time because the only way you will be able to stay within your limits is to eat less, maybe a lot less.

Guess what? You are facing a major lifestyle change. You or your care giver will have to spend a significant amount of time finding something to eat. Also, you will probably have to eat less than you are used to eating. You will also need to limit the amount of fluid you drink. When you first start, it is not a fun time, but it will get easier as you learn and gather information. If you are smart, you will write down what you eat and how much, so you only have to figure it out once.

It's best to avoid canned foods because they generally contain a lot of salt. Always check the label on the can for sodium and potassium.

Deli meats are also an unwise choice because they generally

contain a lot of salt. See an example below.

Deli Roast Beef Nutrition:

Enter Serving Size in Grams 60   Calculate

Water	Protein	Calories	Fat	Carbs	Fiber	Sugars	Phosphorus	Potassium	Sodium
44.22	11.16	69.00	2.22	0.36	0.0	0.18	145.20	388.20	511.80

Values for Phos., Pot., & Sodium are in mg. All others are in grams

60 grams is about two ounces of meat. If you eat deli meat, don't each much of it.

Potato is very high in potassium so keep the portions small or avoid eating potato. Eat rice or pasta instead.

You will also feel better if you eat five or six small meals during the day instead of three. You still need to stay within your limits.

What You Need To Do:

Make a list of the foods you eat regularly.

Meat:

- ground beef,
- beef,
- chicken breast
- pork
- turkey

Vegetables:

- green beans
- peas
- broccoli
- corn
- carrots

Starchy Foods:

- potatoes
- rice
- pasta (all shapes are the same)
- bread
- egg noodles

Fluids:

- water
- milk
- tea
- coffee
- cola

Condiments:

- sugar
- heavy cream
- salt
- Half & Half
- powder Cream Substitute

Put all this information in a spreadsheet like Microsoft Excel with water, protein, phosphorous, potassium and sodium listed on top.

Next, look up the nutrition values on USDA Food Data Central for each item on your list. Copy the data to your spreadsheet. Now you have enough nutrition information to follow a simple diet.

Using the list of regularly eaten foods, I have included nutrition information for each group of foods including meat, vegetables, starchy foods, fluids and condiments. In the following nutrition tables, weight represents serving size. You will probably want to choose different values for serving size.

Meat Nutrition Values:

Item	Weight	Water	Calories	Protein	Fat	Carbs	Fiber	Sugars	Phos.	Pot.	Sodium
Beef, ground, 80% lean meat / 20% fat, patty, cooked, broiled	85	48	230	22	15	0	0	0	165	258	64
Turkey, all classes, light meat, cooked, roasted, serving	85	58	125	26	2	0	0	0	196	212	84
Chicken, Breast, no skin or bone	85	64	92	17	3	0	0	0	168	282	147
Beef, chuck, arm pot roast, separable lean and fat, trimmed to 1/8" fat, choice, cooked, braised, oz	85	42	263	26	17	0	0	0	155	205	42

Vegetable Nutrition Values:

Item	Weight	Water	Calories	Protein	Fat	Carbs	Fiber	Sugars	Phos.	Pot.	Sodium
Peas, Frozen	30	24	23	2	0	4	1	2	25	46	32
Beans, Green, frozen, micro waved	30	27	10	1	0	2	1	1	13	71	1
Broccolli, frozen, cooked, no salt	30	27	8	1	0	2	1	0	17	54	7
Carrots, raw	30	26	12	0	0	3	1	1	11	96	21
Corn, frozen	30	21	34	1	0	8	1	1	28	83	-1

Starchy Food Nutrition Values:

Item	Weight	Water	Calories	Protein	Fat	Carbs	Fiber	Sugars	Phos.	Pot.	Sodium
Bread, white slice, store	30	11	80	3	1	15	1	2	29	38	147
Bread, Homemade White, Panasonic	30	14	68	2	1	13	0	1	21	24	98
Bread, Italian, 1 oz slice	30	11	78	3	1	14	1	1	29	37	185
Bread, wheat, slice	30	11	82	3	1	14	1	2	39	42	142
Noodles, egg cooked	120	81	166	5	2	30	1	0	91	46	6
Rice, white long grain cooked	120	82	156	3	0	34	0	0	52	42	1
Pasta, cooked	120	75	190	7	1	37	2	1	70	53	1
Potatoes, boiled, cooked without skin, flesh, without salt, small (1-3/4" to 2-1/2" dia.)	120	93	103	2	0	24	2	1	48	394	6

Drinks Nutrition Values:

Item	Weight	Water	Calories	Protein	Fat	Carbs	Fiber	Sugars	Phos.	Pot.	Sodium
Water, tap	240	240	0	0	0	0	0	0	0	0	10
Milk; skim	240	218	82	8	0	12	0	12	242	374	101
Tea, brewed; black	240	239	2	0	0	1	0	0	2	89	7
Coffee, brewed, Breakfast Blend; 8 oz	240	239	5	1	0	0	0	0	7	120	2
Soda, cola, regular	240	214	101	0	1	25	0	24	22	12	7

240 grams is equal to 8 ounces or 1 cup.

Condiment Nutrition Values:

Item	Weight	Water	Calories	Protein	Fat	Carbs	Fiber	Sugars	Phos.	Pot.	Sodium
Cream substitute, powdered, cup	5	0	26	0	2	3	0	0	14	33	6
Cream, fluid, half and half, cup	5	4	7	0	1	0	0	0	5	7	3
Cream, heavy whipping	5	3	17	0	2	0	0	0	3	5	1
Sugar, White	5	0	19	0	0	5	0	5	0	0	0
Salt, table	1	0	0	0	0	0	0	0	0	0	342

Don't forget, the weight of a food and protein item is measured in grams while Phosphorous, Potassium and Sodium are measured in milligrams (mg). 1 gram = 1000 mg

5 grams is 1 teaspoon; 1/8 teaspoon of salt weighs .884 grams and gives you 342 mg of sodium; A dash of salt gives you 155 mg of Sodium, so be careful using it. See Chapter 8 for equivalents and other useful information. The easiest thing to do is to make a menu for each day of the week and stick to it for awhile until everything becomes a little easier for you.

The next few pages shows an example of one of my one day meal plans. The example uses the food items I have listed. Hopefully, it will give you a start.

Notice that I have chosen some serving weights. I am not suggesting that you use them, but they are values that worked for me when I first started watching my nutrition. Don't forget that 30 grams equals about 1 ounce. (30g = 1 ounce)

Breakfast Example:

1. 2 large eggs
2. Toast with butter

3. Coffee, 10 oz mug

Sue's Coffee Example:

Item	Weight	Water	Calories	Protein	Fat	Carbs	Fiber	Sugars	Phos.	Pot.	Sodium
Sugar, White	8	0	33	0	0	8	0	8	0	0	0
Cream, heavy whipping	5	3	17	0	2	0	0	0	3	5	1
Coffee, brewed, Breakfast Blend; 8 oz	284	282	6	1	0	0	0	0	9	142	3
Totals	297	285	55	1	2	9	0	9	11	147	4

Please note that I used 10 ounces of coffee, not 8, 1 teaspoon of cream and 2 teaspoons of sugar.

Now that I know the nutrition values for my cup of coffee that I fix the same every time, I can just keep the totals and not have to enter three items each time.

Now I have Sue's coffee listed like the table below:

Sue's Coffee Nutrients:

Serving Size(g) 297   About 10.5 oz.   Recipe Total Weight 297(g) About 10.5 oz.

Water	Calories	Protein	Fat	Carbs	Fiber	Sugars	Phos*	Pot*	Sodium*
285	55	1	2	9	0	9	11	147	4

* Values are in mg. All others are in grams

Now for the rest of breakfast.

Sue's Breakfast

Qty		Item	Weight	Water	Calories	Protein	Fat	Carbs	Fiber	Sugars	Phos.	Pot.	Sodium
2.00	Each	Eggs, large	100	76	143	13	10	1	0	0	198	138	142
1.00	Each	Bread, white slice, store	30	11	80	3	1	15	1	2	29	38	147
1.00	Each	Butter, salted, pat (1" sq, 1/3" high)	5	1	36	0	4	0	0	0	1	1	32
1.00	Serving	Coffee, cream, 2 sugars	297	285	55	1	2	9	0	9	11	147	4
		Totals	432	373	314	17	17	25	1	10	240	324	325

Now for lunch.

Lunch Example:

Sue's Lunch

Qty		Item	Weight	Water	Calories	Protein	Fat	Carbs	Fiber	Sugars	Phos.	Pot.	Sodium
1.00	Each	McDonald's Hamburger	95	42	251	12	10	29	1	6	102	182	469
1.00	Each	McDonald's French Fry, Small	71	26	229	2	11	30	3	0	90	423	134
11.69	Ounce	Soda, Root beer, regular	360	321	148	0	0	38	0	38	0	4	47
		Totals	526	390	628	15	21	97	4	44	192	609	650

Note the high sodium in the hamburger. When you order the hamburger, ask for "no salt."

Also note how high the potassium is and that almost two thirds of it is from the French fries. Potatoes are not a good choice if you are trying to keep your potassium low or maybe only eat half of a small fry.

Let's look at the totals so far.

Daily Log

Item	Weight	Water	Calories	Protein	Fat	Carbs	Fiber	Sugars	Daily Limits 1000 Phos.*	2000 Pot.*	2000 Sodium*
Sue's Breakfast	432.00	373.00	314.00	17.00	16.00	24.00	1.00	11.00	240.00	324.00	325.00
Sue's Lunch	536.00	399.00	632.00	15.00	21.00	98.00	4.00	45.00	192.00	609.00	652.00
Daily Totals	968.00	772.00	946.00	32.00	37.00	122.00	5.00	56.00	432.00	933.00	977.00

| | | | milligrams, all others are in grams | % Daily Totals | 43% | 47% | 49% |

Looks like we are doing OK. We have used up less than half of our nutrition budget. Let's see how we do with supper.

Supper Example:

Now for supper. How about:

1. Pork Pot Roast
2. Potato
3. Green Peas
4. Coffee

Potato twice a day is probably not a good idea, but let's see how it looks. We can always change it.

Supper with Potato

Qty		Item	Weight	Water	Calories	Protein	Fat	Carbs	Fiber	Sugars	Phos.	Pot.	Sodium
1.0	Serving	Pork; Pot Roast	120	90	178	17	12	0	0	0	182	307	59
1.0	Each	Potatoes, boiled, cooked without skin, flesh, without salt, small (1-3/4" to 2-1/2" dia.)	125	97	108	2	0	25	2	1	50	410	6
1.0	Ounce	Peas, Frozen	28.375	23	22	1	0	4	1	1	23	43	31
0.1	Teaspoon	Salt, table	0.4	0	0	0	0	0	0	0	0	0	155
1.0	Serving	Coffee, cream, 2 sugars	297	285	55	1	2	9	0	9	11	147	4
		Totals	571	495	362	21	14	38	4	12	266	908	255

I added a dash of salt for the potato although I don't need it if I use gravy.

Gravy is difficult since I really don't know how much of the nutrients end up in the gravy. Sooo, I assume it is the same as the pot roast. So two tablespoons of gravy at 15 grams each would add 30g to the pot roast weight.

Doesn't look too bad, so let's take a look at the daily totals.

Daily totals with Potato:

Daily Log

Qty	Measure	Item	Weight	Water	Calories	Protein	Fat	Carbs	Fiber	Sugars	Phos.*	Pot.*	Sodium*
											Daily Limits 1000	2000	2000
		Sue's Breakfast	432.00	373.00	314.00	17.00	16.00	24.00	1.00	11.00	240.00	324.00	325.00
		Sue's Lunch	536.00	399.00	632.00	15.00	21.00	98.00	4.00	45.00	192.00	609.00	652.00
		Sue's Supper	566.00	491.00	358.00	20.00	14.00	37.00	3.00	11.00	264.00	892.00	255.00
		Daily Totals	#####	1263.00	1304.00	52.00	51.00	159.00	8.00	67.00	696.00	1825.00	1232.00

*Values are in milligrams, all others are in grams

% Daily Totals	70%	91%	62%

I did good on water; only 1263 grams. Just 263 grams over my limit of one liter. A liter of water is 1000 grams.

I did pretty well considering I had potatoes twice, but I am pretty low on calories, so I really need to eat more. I should give up either the fries for lunch or the potato for supper. Then I could up my calorie count and still stay within my limits. If I ate rice instead of potato, I could probably eat more pot roast.

Let's see what happens when I substitute a cup of rice for the potato in my supper meal.

Supper with Rice

Qty		Item	Weight	Water	Calories	Protein	Fat	Carbs	Fiber	Sugars	Phos.	Pot.	Sodium
1.0	Serving	Pork; Pot Roast	120	90	178	17	12	0	0	0	182	307	59
1.0	Ounce	Peas, Frozen	28.375	23	22	1	0	4	1	1	23	43	31
0.1	Teaspoon	Salt, table	0.4	0	0	0	0	0	0	0	0	0	155
1.0	Serving	Coffee, cream, 2 sugars	297	285	55	1	2	9	0	9	11	147	4
0.76	Cup	Rice, white long grain cooked	120	82	156	3	0	34	0	0	52	42	1
		Totals	566	480	410	22	15	46	2	11	268	540	250

Wow, that really reduced my potassium.

Daily Total with Rice

Daily Log

Qty	Measure	Item	Weight	Water	Calories	Protein	Fat	Carbs	Fiber	Sugars	Phos.*	Pot.*	Sodium*
Date:											1000	2000	2000
		Sue's Breakfast	432.00	373.00	314.00	17.00	16.00	24.00	1.00	11.00	240.00	324.00	325.00
		Sue's Lunch	536.00	399.00	632.00	15.00	21.00	98.00	4.00	45.00	192.00	609.00	652.00
		Sue's Supper with rice	604.00	506.00	460.00	22.00	14.00	58.00	2.00	10.00	284.00	553.00	251.00
		Daily Totals	#####	1278.00	1406.00	54.00	51.00	180.00	7.00	66.00	716.00	1486.00	1228.00

*Values are in milligrams, all others are in grams

% Daily Totals	72%	74%	61%

If I eat rice instead of potato, I can have twice as much pot roast and stay in my nutrition budget. I better not forget about gravy. Rice is pretty bad without anything on it.

If you need a snack, here is the info on a protein bar. There are many different ones available. It would be good if you can find the nutrition information on any bar you buy.

Atkins Cookies n' Crème Bar

Qty		Item	Weight	Water	Calories	Protein	Fat	Carbs	Fiber	Sugars	Phos.	Pot.	Sodium
1.00	Each	Atkins Cookies n' Creme Bar	50.00	0	200	14	11	22	9	1	100	160	200

Part of the adventure into the wilderness of nutrition is finding recipes and their nutrition values. I didn't find it very easy especially since I don't like to cook. I want easy recipes. I've included my recipe for Pork Pot Roast and gravy. It is one of my favorites and I can get my husband to make it. So here it is:

Pork Pot Roast Recipe:

Item	Quantity		Directions
****		CommentLine	Serves 4
Pork, Shoulder, boston butt raw	2	Pound	Add to large fry pan with a tight lid
Pepper, Black ground	1/2	Teaspoon	Add to fry pan
Garlic, Granulated	1/2	Teaspoon	Add to pan
Sage, dry ground	1/2	Teaspoon	Add to fry pan
Marjoram, dried	1	Teaspoon	Add to pan
Water, tap	1	Cup	Add to fry pan; bring to boil; simmer 2 hrs;
****		CommentLine	Add water as necessary; bottom of pan should always be covered
****		CommentLine	Remove pork from pan; place on a platter; set aside
****		CommentLine	

Pork Pot Roast Nutrients:

Serving Size(g) 120   About 4.2 oz.   Recipe Total Weight 1,145(g) About 40.4 oz.

Water	Calories	Protein	Fat	Carbs	Fiber	Sugars	Phos*	Pot*	Sodium*
90	178	17	12	0	0	0	182	307	59

*Values are in mg. All others are in grams

The above values are for a serving size of about four ounces.

Here is the recipe for pork pot roast gravy that I use.

Pork Pot Roast Gravy Recipe:

Item	Quantity		Directions
****		CommentLine	Makes about 4 cups of gravy
Soup, stock, beef, home-prepared, cup	1	Cup	Put meat on a platter. Pour liquid from pot roast pan into 4 cup Pyrex measure
Water, tap	2	Cup	Add water to make 3 cups; stir and return to fry pan on low heat
Flour, All Purpose	4	Tablespoon	Add flour to pint shaker jar with lid
Water, tap	1	Cup	Add water to flour in shaker jar; replace lid shake until all flour is mixed
****		CommentLine	Whisk flour mixture into fry pan; mix well
Sage, dry ground	1/2	Teaspoon	Add to fry pan;
Marjoram, dried	1/2	Teaspoon	Add to fry pan; mix well
****		CommentLine	Cook on medium heat; Stir constantly with spatula until thick; simmer for 2 more min. Serve
****		CommentLine	Add water if too thick; Add flour water mixture if too thin

Pork Pot Roast Gravy Nutrients:

Serving Size(g) 120   About 4.2 oz.   Recipe Total Weight 973(g) About 34.3 oz.

Water	Calories	Protein	Fat	Carbs	Fiber	Sugars	Phos*	Pot*	Sodium*
115	18	1	0	3	0	0	13	60	62

*Values are in mg. All others are in grams

This serving would be about ½ cup of gravy.

Some of you may be wondering how we got these nice recipes and charts. A long story short. I am a software developer and when I had to start following my kidney diet, I designed and wrote software for a food database. It contains everything that I eat, including all our recipes; it also includes nutrition tracking software. It was a life saver when I went on dialysis, especially when I first started and was in a dialysis center.

I really want to help those of you who are struggling to figure out what to eat and how to get the information you need. I struggled for weeks getting the information I needed when I first started.

When I got fed up struggling to use the USDA Data Central food database, I wrote a software app to make it much, much easier to get the information I needed. The app is called the KDC Food Finder which I am making available to anyone who wants to use it for a small fee. Included with the application are several spreadsheets that make nutrition much easier to track.

Processed Foods and Shopping

I have nothing good to say about processed foods except "don't eat them." If you want to be successful in following a kidney diet, stop eating processed foods. In general, they are full of sodium and phosphorous. There might be processed foods that won't bust your nutrition budget, but I have not found many, nor have I looked very hard.

The first rule of shopping is to carefully read the food labels on everything including meats. Read and understand them. Understanding them is the hard part.

The label always gives you a serving weight in grams and sometimes a volume like a cup. It also gives you weights of sodium, potassium and protein. It seldom gives you the value of phosphorous.

For example, I am looking at a can of red kidney beans. The serving size is listed as ½ cup or 130 grams.

Sodium is listed on the label as 130 mg (milligrams). You get 130 mg of sodium if you eat 130g of beans. Easy so far.

Potassium is listed as 340 mg for every 130g of beans you eat. OK so far.

Phosphorous is not listed as it is not required to be put on the label. Strike out. What do I do now? You go to USDA Food Data Central and try to find out how much phosphorous you are eating.

Do I have to? The answer to that question is another question. How important is it to you to track your nutrition? Remember what you read about phosphorous in chapter 1.

If it is too high, it can cause calcified organs, weakened bones, bone pain, itching, and muscle weakness. If it is too low, it can cause appetite loss and confusion. Consider the consequences of not paying attention to Phosphorous. Then decide if you are going forward or giving up.

To find out how much phosphorous there is in kidney beans go to USDA Food Data Central to get the information or use KDC Food Finder. Using KDC Food Finder is much easier. As illustrated on the next page.

You can access the KDC Food Finder here:
 https://kidneyfoodfinder.com.

You can find Food Data Central here: https://fdc.nal.usda.gov.

Kidney Bean Nutrition:

| Beans, kidney, red, mature seeds, canned, s ⌄ | Choose |

Nutrients per Gram of (USDA # 175195)
Beans, kidney, red, mature seeds, canned, solids and liquids

Water	0.780	g
Protein	0.052	g
Calories	0.810	kcal
Fat	0.004	g
Carbs	0.148	g
Fiber	0.043	g
Sugars	0.019	g
Phosphorus	1.060	mg
Potassium	2.600	mg
Sodium	2.560	mg

Grams per Unit of Measure

Qty	Item	Grams
1	can	436
1	tbsp	16
1	cup	256

Enter Serving Size in Grams 10   Calculate

Water	Protein	Calories	Fat	Carbs	Fiber	Sugars	Phosphorus	Potassium	Sodium
7.80	0.52	8.10	0.04	1.48	0.43	0.19	10.60	26.00	25.60

Values for Phos., Pot., & Sodium are in mg. All others are in grams

Note that the values listed in the first chart are for 1 gram of kidney beans. See below for a serving size of 130 grams.

Grams per Unit of Measure

Qty	Item	Grams
1	can	436
1	tbsp	16
1	cup	256

Enter Serving Size in Grams 130   [Calculate]

Water	Protein	Calories	Fat	Carbs	Fiber	Sugars	Phosphorus	Potassium	Sodium
101.40	6.76	105.30	0.52	19.24	5.59	2.47	137.80	338.00	332.80

Values for Phos., Pot., & Sodium are in mg. All others are in grams

Using the data from the tables above, I get 137mg of phosphorous in a 130gram serving of Kidney beans which is 13.7 percent of my daily phosphorous budget. To me this can be significant. Is this worth looking up? It is to me, how else am I going to keep my phosphorous under control? If I keep the information in a spreadsheet, I don't have to look it up again.

If you are paying close attention you will notice that the Sodium is listed on the label of the can of kidney beans is 130 mg (milligrams). The Sodium listed on the USDA data sheet is 332 mg. Why are the numbers for sodium so different?

I have no idea how much salt was used to prepare this can of kidney beans. It appears to be much less than the average can of kidney beans. This highlights how important it is to read food labels.

Phosphates are used as preservatives in many foods. Look at the ingredient list for any word with "phos" in it. Look for potassium too. Phosphates are more easily absorbed by the body than naturally occurring phosphorous.

There is not much processed food you buy in a store that will have phosphorous information on the label. So be careful.

Meats:

Be careful when you buy meats, especially chicken, turkey and pork. A lot of grocery store meat, including pork, turkey, chicken and sometimes beef are injected with a saline solution. The solution usually includes water and other ingredients such as salt, phosphates, antioxidants, and flavorings. The reason given for this process is to improve juiciness, tenderness and flavor, and to extend the shelf-life. This is called enhanced meat.

According to Wikipedia, Plumped chicken (enhanced chicken) commonly contains 15% of its total weight in saltwater. It is not uncommon to see solutions of 10 to 15 percent added to meat.

Watch out for words like basted, injected, enhanced and marinated. These words are a warning that meat has been injected with something that is not healthy for someone on a kidney diet. Non-enhanced meat contains no added salt, solutions or flavorings.

Look for fancy packages with recognizable brand names that use phrases like always tender, moist and juicy, tender and juicy, Then look for the fine print: *Solution ingredients: Water, salt, sodium phosphates or something similar.

Retail Pork products are often injected with a 7% to 12% solution which most often contains water, sodium lactate, sodium phosphates, potassium lactate, and/or sodium diacetate.

I don't know about you, but I don't need the extra, water, salt, phosphorous or potassium in my diet.

When you buy a pound of enhanced meat at $5 a pound, you will be getting 14 ounces of meat and 2 ounces of salt water. This brings the price of the actual meat up to $5.71 per pound.

For more information see my blog on kidney diet tips. https://kidneydietcentral.com/blog

Home Cooking:

Home cooking is the name of the game and is your best chance of meeting you nutrition budget. The second part of the game is to throw out your salt shaker. Don't use salt. This takes some getting used to. After a while, any prepared food you buy in the store will taste salty.

Instead of salt, I use garlic powder (not garlic salt). It doesn't take much to make a difference in taste and it does help lessen your need for salt.

Let me give you an example. Here is a comparison of my homemade white bread versus store bought white bread.

Homemade White Bread vs Store Bought White Bread.

Qty		Item	Weight	Water	Calories	Protein	Fat	Carbs	Fiber	Sugars	Phos.	Pot.	Sodium
1.00	Each	Bread, white slice, store	30.00	11	80	3	1	15	1	2	29	38	147
0.52	Serving	Bread, Homemade White, Panasonic	30	14	68	2	1	13	0	1	21	24	98
		Totals	60	25	148	4	2	28	1	2	51	61	245

The difference in sodium is almost 50mg (milligrams) for one slice of bread. For a whole sandwich it is nearly 100mg which makes room for more homemade roast beef.

There is a catch. My husband Bill revised the original recipe that came with the bread machine and reduced the salt by one half. See his recipe in the Chapter 7, recipes.

Chili powder is another surprising source of salt.

Chili Powder Comparison:

Item	Weight	Water	Calories	Protein	Fat	Carbs	Fiber	Sugars	Phos.	Pot.	Sodium
Chili Powder, purchased	8.	1	23	1	1	4	3	1	24	156	229
Chili Powder, Homemade	8	1	26	1	1	5	2	0	29	129	6

A weight of 8 grams is about a teaspoon. I showed you this chart to show you the importance of reading labels. 143 milligrams is a lot of sodium.

Eating Out:

Once I found out how closely I had to watch my diet, I didn't eat out until I got to know how to choose foods I could eat. Fish fry for example. I can get nutrient values for fried fish, French fries and coleslaw directly from USDA Food Data Central.

Here is an example of nutrition numbers for a typical restaurant fish fry.

Fish Fry Dinner Nutrition:

Qty		Item	Weight	Water	Calories	Protein	Fat	Carbs	Fiber	Sugars	Phos.	Pot.	Sodium
1.00	Cup	Cabbage, raw, cup, shredded	70.00	65	18	1	0	4	2	2	18	119	13
2.00	Tablespoon	Salad dressing, coleslaw, tbsp	38	15	154	0	13	9	0	8	16	13	323
1.00	Each	Restaurant, family style, fish fillet, battered or breaded, fried, serving	226.00	128	495	30	24	38	2	1	468	567	1268
1.00	Each	Restaurant, family style, french fries, serving	170.00	73	491	6	24	63	7	0	211	927	607
		Totals	504	282	1157	36	62	114	11	11	713	1626	2211

These are not nice numbers if you are on a kidney diet. I will try again and eat only half as much this time.

Qty		Item	Weight	Water	Calories	Protein	Fat	Carbs	Fiber	Sugars	Phos.	Pot.	Sodium
.5	Cup	Cabbage, raw, cup, shredded	35	32	9	0	0	2	1	1	9	60	6
1	Tablespoon	Salad dressing, coleslaw, tbsp	19	8	77	0	7	4	0	4	8	7	162
.5	Each	Restaurant, family style, fish fillet, battered or breaded, fried, serving	113	64	247	15	12	19	1	1	234	284	634
.5	Each	Restaurant, family style, french fries, serving	85	37	246	3	12	32	3	0	105	463	303
		Totals	252	140	578	18	31	67	6	6	357	812	1106

Much better results this time. Portion Control is the name of the game.

When I first went on dialysis, actually before I started on dialysis, I carried a small scale with me so I could know how much I was eating. I even carried a paper plate in my purse, so I had a plate to put on my scale. Some restaurants will give you an extra plate so it is easier to re-portion your meal.

It's a good idea to know what you are going to eat before you walk into a restaurant. That way you can be prepared to control your portion and not bust you daily budget too badly. Using the chart above for a fish fry, you can eat in a restaurant and know how much fish, fries and slaw you can eat without breaking your nutrition budget.

It is difficult to find information on restaurant food and that is why I didn't eat out until I got to know food I could eat. Even if you do find information on restaurant food, you don't know how well it represents the food at the restaurant at which you are eating. Some cooks are much heavier handed with salt than others and remember a dash of salt is worth 155mg of sodium. This is one of the reasons I chose not to eat out until my labs and diet were under control.

I have added a steak dinner and a pork chop dinner to give you an idea of what to expect. Some steak houses add seasonings to their steak which often include salt. You may want to order a steak with no seasonings.

These two dinners plus the fish fry will help get you started tracking your diet while eating out.

Steak Dinner Nutrition:

Qty		Item	Weight	Water	Calories	Protein	Fat	Carbs	Fiber	Sugars	Phos.	Pot.	Sodium
4.00	Ounce	Beef, top sirloin, steak, broiled, separable lean and fat, trimmed to 1/8	113	86	276	31	16	0	0	0	237	381	64
0.49	Cup	Potatoes, baked, flesh, without salt, cup	60	45	56	1	0	13	1	1	30	235	3
1.08	Ounce	Sour cream, imitation, cultured, oz	30	21	62	1	6	2	0	2	14	48	31
1.00	Each	McDonald's Side Salad	87	82	17	1	0	4	1	2	17	191	10
1.00	Each	Salad dressing, ranch dressing, regular, tablespoon	15	7	65	0	7	1	0	1	28	10	135
1.01	Ounce	Whiskey, 86 proof	30	19	75	0	0	0	0	0	1	0	0
1.00	Ounce	Soda, Ginger ale	31	28	10	0	0	3	0	3	0	0	2
		Totals	366	268	561	34	29	23	2	9	327	865	246

Not bad, especially low on salt unless you salt your steak or use steak sauce. Remember to order your steak with no salt! Don't forget, a dash of salt is 155mg of sodium. It looks like you can afford a couple of dashes of salt with this meal. You even get to have a mixed drink.

You probably noticed that I used a McDonald's side salad. There were not many choices in the database, and this is about the right size. It is absolutely a best guess and you have to use information that you can find and use it as a guideline.

A pork chop makes a decent meal, but not as good as a beef steak meal if you remembered to ask for a steak with no seasoning. A pork chop will probably be seasoned as well, so ask your server about that too.

Pork Chop Dinner Nutrition:

Qty		Item	Weight	Water	Calories	Protein	Fat	Carbs	Fiber	Sugars	Phos.	Pot.	Sodium
1.0	Ounce	Whiskey, 86 proof	30	19	75	0	0	0	0	0	1	0	0
1.0	Ounce	Soda, Ginger ale, regular	30.5	28	10	0	0	3	0	3	0	0	2
1.0	Each	McDonald's Side Salad	87	82	17	1	0	4	1	2	17	191	10
1.0	Each	Salad dressing, ranch dressing, regular, tablespoon	15	7	65	0	7	1	0	1	28	10	135
0.7	Each	Pork, fresh, center loin (chops), bone-in, pan-fried	120	70	286	33	16	0	0	0	301	424	113
0.5	Cup	Potatoes, baked, flesh, without salt, cup	60	45	56	1	0	13	1	1	30	235	3
1.1	Ounce	Sour cream, imitation, cultured, oz	30	21	62	1	6	2	0	2	14	48	31
		Totals	373	272	571	37	29	23	2	9	392	909	294

Not bad again, but remember you are not eating a whole pork chop or a whole potato. Portion control, there is that word again. I know you hate to hear it, but at least you get to eat a good meal and something you like.

The problem with this diet thing is that it is takes so long to find out how well you are doing. You have to stick to a diet and wait for your labs to become available. Your lab results are like your report card. If the numbers are within the normal range, you are doing well with your diet. If not, you need to change your diet. This whole deal is not easy or fun, but it is doable. If you do it, you will feel better for your troubles.

Chapter 6: Recipes

I have included many of our recipes that I used all the time I was on dialysis and they all include the nutrition information you need to make good choices.

BEWARE: These recipes are not all kidney diet friendly. Be sure to read the nutrition information before you decide what you are going to eat and adjust your portion size accordingly.

Above all, practice **PORTION CONTROL**. You can eat anything in this list as long as you don't eat too much of it.

I show serving size on each recipe. I am not suggesting that this is the right serving size for you, it is just a place to start. Adjust the portion sizes to fit your needs.

Don't Forget: **don't add salt**.

Beef and Peppers

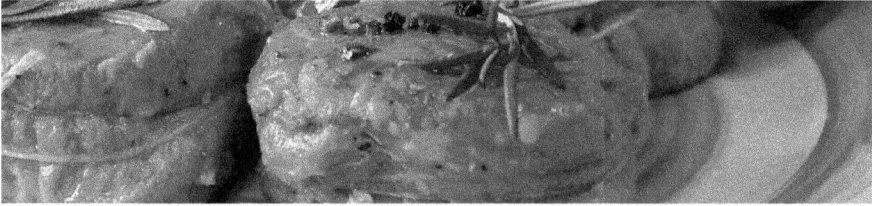

Item	Quantity		Directions
****	CommentLine		Makes 5 servings; about 8 ounces (217 gram) each
Bouillon Cube, Beef	1	Each	add 1 cube to 1 cup glass measure
Water, tap	1	Cup	Add to cup; cook in microwave on high for 4 min; stir until dissolved
****	CommentLine		Add to large fry pan
Mushrooms, white, raw	2	Cup	Mushrooms sliced, Add to fry pan
Peppers, Bell raw, sliced	1	Cup	Slice peppers 1/2 inch wide and 1 inch long; Add to fry pan
Onion; medium; 110g	1	Each	medium onion sliced thin, Add to fry pan
Beef, Round, raw	1/2	Pound	Slice thin and cut 1 inch long. Add to fry pan
Pepper, Black ground	1/4	Teaspoon	Add to fry pan
Ginger, Ground	1	Teaspoon	Add to fry pan
Worcestershire Sauce	1	Tablespoon	Add to fry pan
Sugar, White	1	Tablespoon	Add to fry pan
Basil, dried leaves	1	Teaspoon	Add to fry pan; mix
****	CommentLine		Cover pan; Simmer 6 min on medium heat
Cornstarch	2	Tablespoon	Add to shaker jar
Water, tap	1	Cup	Add to shaker jar; shake well
****	CommentLine		Slowly add to fry pan; stir constantly
****	CommentLine		Stir constantly until thick; add water if necessary
****	CommentLine		

Comments

Serve with rice or egg noodles

Serving Size(g) 218 About 7.7 oz. Recipe Total Weight 1,089(g) About 38.4 oz.

Water	Calories	Protein	Fat	Carbs	Fiber	Sugars	Phos*	Pot*	Sodium*
189	135	11	6	10	1	5	131	350	264

*Values are in mg. All others are in grams

Beef Stew

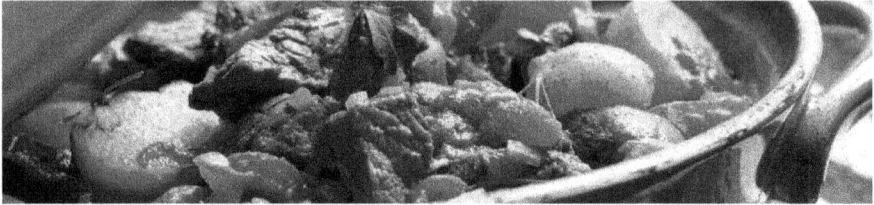

Item	Quantity		Directions
****		CommentLine	Makes8 servings, 8ounce (226 gram) each
Beef, Chuck	1 1/2	Pound	Cut into 3/4 inch cubes; place in crock pot
Water, tap	1/2	Cup	Add to pot
Potatoes, white, boiled,no skin	8	Ounce	Peel 3 small potatoes, cut in half; add to pot
Onion; medium; 110g	1/2	Each	2 to 2 1/2 inch onion; Slice 1/4 thick; Add to pot
Mushrooms, white, raw	4	Ounce	slice, 6 medium mushrooms, add to pot.
Thyme, dried Leaves	1/2	Teaspoon	Add to pot
Marjoram, dried	1/2	Teaspoon	Add to pot
Parsley, dried	1/2	Teaspoon	Add to pot
Peppers, Bell, raw chopped	4	Ounce	Dice,1 medium pepper; Add to pot
Garlic, Minced	1/2	Teaspoon	Add to pot;
Pepper, Black ground	1/2	Teaspoon	Add to pot; Cook on LO for 6-8 hours
****		CommentLine	When stew is cooked, pour liquid into a 1 qt Pyrex cup
Water, tap	1	Cup	Add water to cup to make 2 cups of broth; Set aside
Flour, All Purpose	5	Tablespoon	Add flour to shaking jar (16 ounce jar with a lid)
Salt, table	1/8	Teaspoon	Add 1/8 teaspoon salt to to shaking jar
Water, tap	1	Cup	Add water to shaking jar; tighten lid and shake till flour dissolved
****		CommentLine	Add to Pyrex cup. Cook in microwave for 1 minute on HI
****		CommentLine	Mix well. Repeat until thick. Add water if too thicken
****		CommentLine	Cook for 3 minutes on power level 5; Return gravy to pot or serve separately

Comments

A Medium onion is 2-2½ inches in diameter and weighs about 110 gm. Good with rice or egg noodles. Good on biscuits except for the extra salt.

Serving Size(g) 226   About 8 oz.   Recipe Total Weight 1,817(g) About 64.1 oz.

Water	Calories	Protein	Fat	Carbs	Fiber	Sugars	Phos*	Pot*	Sodium*
165	209	18	10	11	1	1	192	446	115

Values are in mg. All others are in grams

Beef and Vegetables

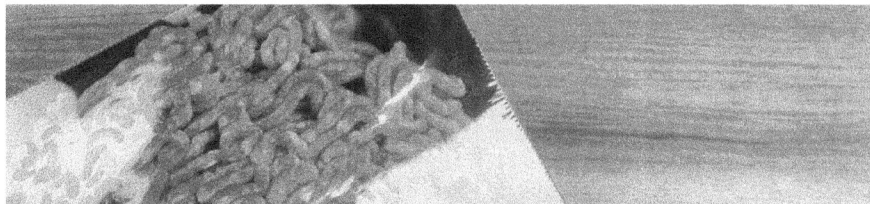

Item		Quantity	Directions
****		CommentLine	Makes 5 servings, about 8 ounces each
Beef, Ground 80%, raw	1	Pound	Crumble and add to large fry pan
Thyme, dried Leaves	2	Teaspoon	Add to fry pan
Garlic, Minced	2	Teaspoon	Add to fry pan
****		CommentLine	Cook beef until done
Corn, frozen	1	Cup	Add to fry pan
Peas, Frozen	1	Cup	Add to fry pan
Mushrooms, white, raw	1	Cup	Slice mushrooms and add to fry pan
Onion; medium, 110g	1	Cup	slice onion 1/4 inch thick and quarter, Add to fry pan
Water, tap	1	Cup	Add to fry pan
****		CommentLine	simmer until onions are tender about 5 minutes
****		CommentLine	
****		CommentLine	
****		CommentLine	

Comments

Serve with rice or egg noodles; Also good on biscuits except they are much more salty.

Serving Size(g) 240   About 8.5 oz.   Recipe Total Weight 1,199(g) About 42.3 oz.

Water	Calories	Protein	Fat	Carbs	Fiber	Sugars	Phos*	Pot*	Sodium*
185	304	19	19	15	3	4	219	471	95

* Values are in mg. All others are in grams

Beef, Roast

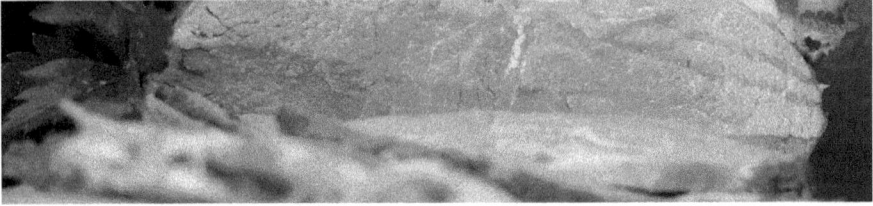

Item		Quantity	Directions
****		CommentLine	Makes about 12, four ounce (120 grams) servings
Beef, Round, raw	3	Pound	Place in glass baking dish
Thyme, dried Leaves	1	Teaspoon	Spread on beef and bottom of pan
Marjoram, dried	1	Teaspoon	Spread on beef and bottom of pan
Pepper, Black ground	1/4	Teaspoon	Spread on beef and bottom of pan
Garlic, Granulated	1/2	Teaspoon	Spread on beef and bottom of pan
Parsley, dried	1	Teaspoon	Spread on beef and bottom of pan
****		CommentLine	Cook in 325° oven to 150°F, about 3 hrs
****		CommentLine	To make gravy: Put meat on a platter and then
New Item	1	CommentLine	Pour liquid from pot roast pan into 4 cup measure;
****		CommentLine	To make gravy, follow separate recipe for roast beef gravy

Comments

Makes great sandwiches with some mayo and horseradish -- see recipe for roast beef sandwich

Serving Size(g) 120   About 4.2 oz.   Recipe Total Weight 1,365(g) About 48.2 oz.

Water	Calories	Protein	Fat	Carbs	Fiber	Sugars	Phos*	Pot*	Sodium*
78	234	25	14	0	0	0	239	414	65

* Values are in mg. All others are in grams

Beef, Roast Beef Sandwich, Deli Beef

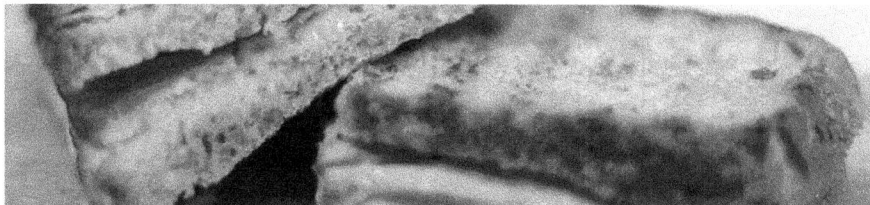

Item		Quantity	Directions
Bread, white slice, store	2	Each	
Mayonnaise, Light	1	Tablespoon	Spread evenly on both slices of bread
Horseradish, prepared	1	Tablespoon	Spread evenly on one slice of bread
Roast beef, deli style, prepackaged, sliced. slice oval	3	Ounce	Place evenly on hrseradish piece of bread
Lettuce, iceburg	18	Gram	Place on top of beef
****		CommentLine	Place second slice of bread on top of beef. Enjoy

Comments

Notice the large amount of sodium and potassium in deli beef.

Serving Size(g) 193   About 6.8 oz.   Recipe Total Weight 193(g) About 6.8 oz.

Water	Calories	Protein	Fat	Carbs	Fiber	Sugars	Phos*	Pot*	Sodium*
124	303	22	9	34	2	6	275	693	1,208

*Values are in mg. All others are in grams

I included a roast beef sandwich made with deli meat so you could see what a bad choice deli meat is. See the following page for a sandwich make with home cooked roast beef.

Beef, Roast Beef Sandwich, homemade beef

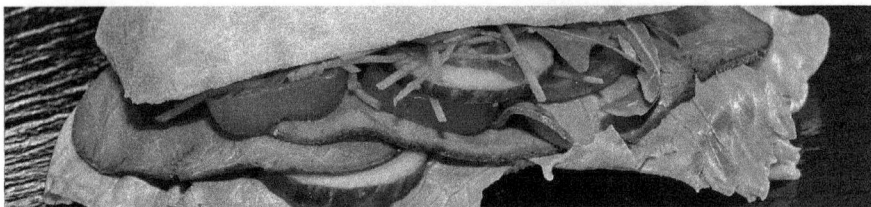

Item	Quantity		Directions
****	CommentLine		Makes 1 sandwich
Bread, Homemade White, Panasonic	1	Each	Cut bread in half
Mayonnaise, Light	1	Tablespoon	Spread evenly on both slices of bread
Horseradish, prepared	1	Tablespoon	Spread evenly on one slice of bread
Beef, Roast, homemade	3	Ounce	Place evenly on bread
Lettuce, iceburg	18	Gram	Place on top of beef
****		CommentLine	Place second slice of bread on top of beef, enjoy

Comments

Hight in phosphorous, potassium and sodium

Serving Size(g) 191   About 6.7 oz.   Recipe Total Weight 191(g) About 6.7 oz.

Water	Calories	Protein	Fat	Carbs	Fiber	Sugars	Phos*	Pot*	Sodium*
123	343	21	15	29	2	3	221	406	425

* Values are in mg. All others are in grams

Beef, Teriyaki Beef and Peppers

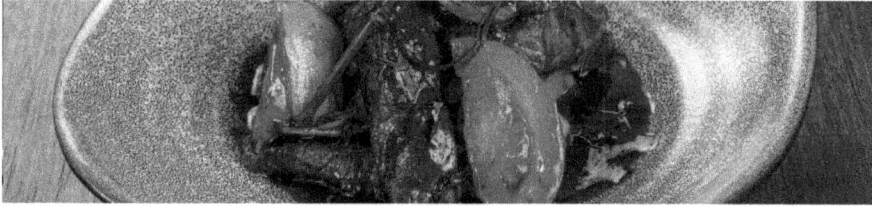

Item	Quantity		Directions
****		CommentLine	makes 4 six ounce (182 gm) servings
Teriyaki Sauce	1	Each	Make Teriyaki Sauce; set aside
Oil, Canola	1	Tablespoon	add to fry pan;
Beef, top sirloin, steak, raw, separable lean and fat, trimmed to 1/8	1	Pound	Cut beef into 1/4; add to frypan; saute on medium heat
Peppers, Bell raw, sliced	1	Cup	Add to fry pan
Onion; medium; 110g	1	Each	Add to fry pan; saute until peppers are tender
****	1	CommentLine	Add Teriyaki sauce to frypan; simmer 5 minutes
****		CommentLine	Serve over rice

Comments

Serve with Rice

Serving Size(g) 182   About 6.4 oz.   Recipe Total Weight 730(g) About 25.7 oz.

Water	Calories	Protein	Fat	Carbs	Fiber	Sugars	Phos*	Pot*	Sodium*
125	277	24	18	4	1	2	225	439	74

* Values are in mg. All others are in grams

Bread, White Homemade Bread

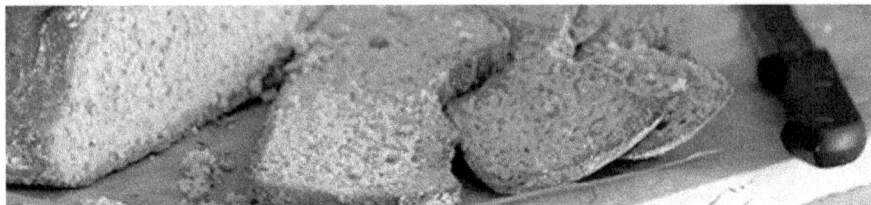

Item	Quantity		Directions
****		CommentLine	Recipe is for Panasonic Bread maker; Makes 15 slices, about 2 oz (55g) each
Flour, All Purpose	3 3/4	Cup	Add to breadmaker pan
Salt, table	1	Teaspoon	Add to bread pan
Milk, Dry Instant Non Fat, A&D	2	Tablespoon	Add to bread pan
Butter	2	Tablespoon	Add to bread pan
Sugar, White	1	Tablespoon	Add to bread pan
Water, tap	1 1/2	Cup	Add to bread pan, place pan in bread maker
Yeast, baker's, Dry	1	Teaspoon	Add to yeast dispenser
****		CommentLine	Set bread maker to: Basic, Large, Light
****		CommentLine	Takes 4 hours to finish

Comments

Kidney friendly-- Makes a sizable, tall loaf -- 15 slices, about 55 grams each -- 1 slice cut in half is about the same size of a slice of store sandwich bread

Serving Size(g) 55   About 2 oz.   Recipe Total Weight 879(g) About 31 oz.

Water	Calories	Protein	Fat	Carbs	Fiber	Sugars	Phos*	Pot*	Sodium*
27	132	4	2	25	1	1	41	46	190

* Values are in mg. All others are in grams

Chicken Stir Fry with General Toas Sauce

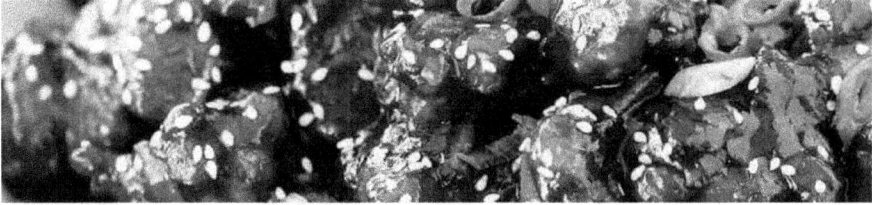

Item		Quantity	Directions
****		CommentLine	Makes about 4 servings, 9 ounces (262gm) each
****		CommentLine	Prepare recipe for Gen Toas Sauce; set aside
Chicken, Breast, no skin or bone	1	Pound	Slice 1/4 thick, then cut into 1 inch squares; set aside
Onion; medium; 110g	1	Each	Slice 1/4 thick; cut slices in half; set aside
Peppers; Bell, raw chopped	1/2	Cup	Slice into 1/4 inch strips; set aside
Celery, raw, cup chopped	1/2	Cup	Chop 1 large (11-12) stalk 1/4 inch thick; cut in half, set aside
Vegetables, frozen, mixed	5	Ounce	Thaw 1/2 10 oz package of oriental veggies; set aside
****	2	Tablespoon	Add to large fry pan; place over medium heat
****		CommentLine	Add chicken to pan; saute on medium heat until chicken is cooked; push aside
****	1	Tablespoon	Add to bare part of fry pan
****		CommentLine	Add Onions, peppers, celery and mixed veggies to fry pan; Saute for 5 minutes
Gen Toas Sauce	1	Cup	Add to fry pan, simmer for 5 minutes on medium heat. Serve over rice
****		CommentLine	New recipe

Comments

Serve with rice

Serving Size(g) 262   About 9.2 oz.   Recipe Total Weight 1,048(g) About 37 oz.

Water	Calories	Protein	Fat	Carbs	Fiber	Sugars	Phos*	Pot*	Sodium*
212	211	25	4	18	3	9	269	589	435

*Values are in mg. All others are in grams

Gen Toas Sauce is our version of Gen Tso Sauce.

Corn Bread

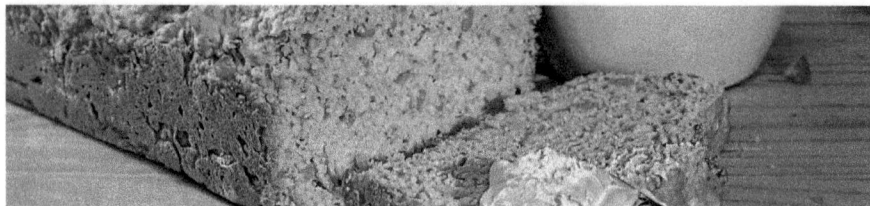

Item	Quantity		Directions
****		CommentLine	Makes about 10 servings, 2 ounces each
Flour, All Purpose	1 1/4	Cup	Add to 4 cup bowl
Cornmeal; yellow	3/4	Cup	Add to bowl
Sugar, White	1/3	Cup	Add to bowl
Baking Powder	2	Teaspoon	Add to bowl
Salt, table	1/8	Teaspoon	Add to bowl; combine
Milk; skim	1	Cup	Add to bowl
Oil, Canola	2	Tablespoon	Add to bowl
Eggs, large	1	Each	Add to bowl; mix well
****		CommentLine	Pour into a lightly Pamed 11 x 7 baking dish
****		CommentLine	Bake at 400°F for 20-25 minutes till golden brown

Comments

Oh, so good! It doesn't last long in our house/

Serving Size(g) 60   About 2.1 oz.   Recipe Total Weight 647(g) About 22.8 oz.

Water	Calories	Protein	Fat	Carbs	Fiber	Sugars	Phos*	Pot*	Sodium*
27	145	4	3	25	1	7	87	82	140

* Values are in mg. All others are in grams

Fish, Baked Haddock

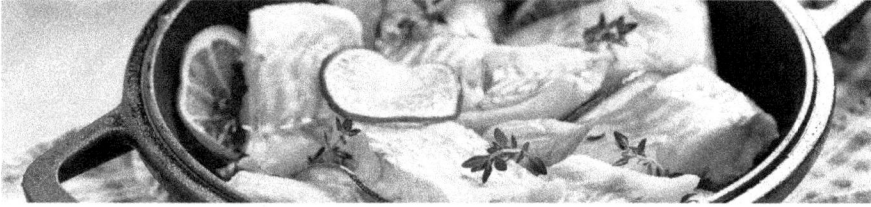

Item	Quantity		Directions
****		CommentLine	Makes two small servings, about 4.5 ounces each
Fish, Haddock, raw	8	Ounce	Place in glass baking dish
Butter	1	Tablespoon	Melt butter; spread evenly on fish
Garlic, Granulated	1/8	Teaspoon	Spread evenly on fish
Pepper, Black ground	1/8	Teaspoon	Add pepper to taste; Spread evenly on fish
Oregano	1/8	Teaspoon	Spread evenly on fish
Lemon Juice	1	Tablespoon	Spread evenly on fish
****		CommentLine	Bake at 350°F for 35 minutes; or microwave 2 minutes at power level 5
****		CommentLine	

Comments

The garlic, pepper, oregano and lemon juice can be mixed with the melted butter and the combination spread evenly on the fish.

Serving Size(g) 128   About 4.5 oz.   Recipe Total Weight 257(g) About 9.1 oz.

Water	Calories	Protein	Fat	Carbs	Fiber	Sugars	Phos*	Pot*	Sodium*
102	137	19	6	1	0	0	260	339	288

* Values are in mg. All others are in grams

Hamburg and Gravy

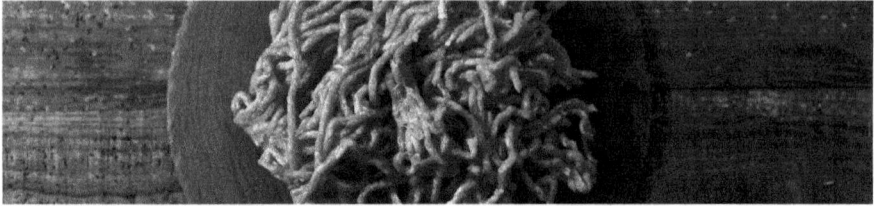

Item	Quantity		Directions
****		CommentLine	Makes about 2 servings, with 4 ounces (117 gm) of meat each. Plus 2 Tbl gravy
Beef, Ground 80%, raw	8	Ounce	Crumble & Cook in 10 inch fry pan until done
Water, tap	1 1/2	Cup	Add to fry pan and stir
Pepper, Black ground	1/2	Teaspoon	Add to fry pan
Thyme, dried Leaves	1	Teaspoon	Add to fry pan
Garlic, Granulated	1	Teaspoon	Add to fry pan
Salt, table	1/4	Teaspoon	Add to fry pan and stir
Flour, All Purpose	3	Tablespoon	Add flour to pint jar with top
Water, tap	1	Cup	Add water to jar, Cover jar and shake until flour is all mixed.
****		CommentLine	Slowly add to fry pan wisking constantly. Simmer 5 minutes. Add water if necessary

Comments

Good over egg noodles or rice. Good on toast or biscuits but they add extra salt-- Don't forget . Do not cook rice or noodles in salted water. n ---Serving size includes 2 tablespoons of gravy

Serving Size(g) 141   About 5 oz.   Recipe Total Weight 840(g) About 29.6 oz.

Water	Calories	Protein	Fat	Carbs	Fiber	Sugars	Phos*	Pot*	Sodium*
122	113	7	8	3	0	0	67	116	140

* Values are in mg. All others are in grams

Hamburg and Gravy with Vegetables

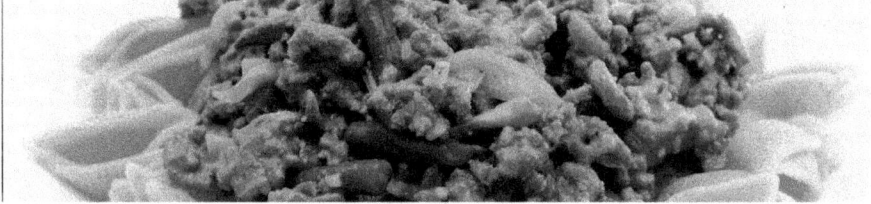

Item	Quantity		Directions
****		CommentLine	Makes about 6 servings; 8 ounces (227 gm) each
Beef, Ground 80%, raw	1	Pound	Add to large fry pan, crumble and cook
Corn, frozen	1	Cup	Add to large fry pan
Onion, medium, 110g	1	Each	Dice onion and add to pan
Peppers, Bell, raw chopped	1/2	Each	Add to pan
Water, tap	1	Cup	Use pyrex measuring cup
Bouillon Cube, Beef	1	Each	Add to pyrex cup; microwave on hi for 4 min; stir add to fry pan
Thyme, dried Leaves	1	Teaspoon	Add to fry pan
Marjoram, dried	1	Teaspoon	Add to fry pan
Parsley, dried	1	Teaspoon	Add to fry pan
Garlic, Granulated	1	Teaspoon	Add to fry pan
Pepper, Black ground	1/2	Teaspoon	Add to fry pan
Fennel seed	1/4	Teaspoon	add ground fennel seed to fry pan
****		CommentLine	Simmer for 6 to 8 min until pepper is cooked
Water, tap	1	Cup	Add to fry pan , mix
Flour, All Purpose	3	Tablespoon	Add flour to shaker jar
Water, tap	1	Cup	Add to shaker jar; shake until flour disolved;
****		CommentLine	Slowly add to fry pan while stiring briskly; simmer 3 minutes until thick
****		CommentLine	New Recipe; not tried 10/7/15

Comments

Serve over egg noodles, rice or pasta. Remember, don't cook them in salted water.

Serving Size(g) 240   About 8.5 oz.   Recipe Total Weight 1,439(g) About 50.7 oz.

Water	Calories	Protein	Fat	Carbs	Fiber	Sugars	Phos*	Pot*	Sodium*
197	245	15	16	12	1	2	157	317	213

Values are in mg. All others are in grams

Macaroni and Cheese

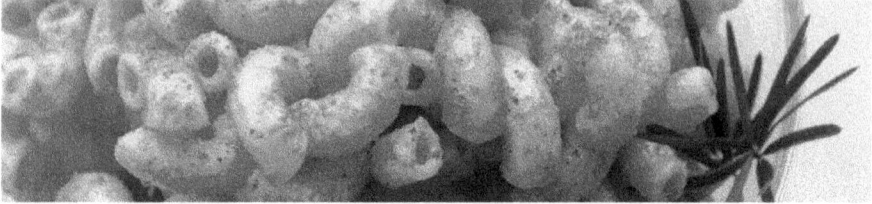

Item		Quantity		Directions
****			CommentLine	Makes about 8 servings, 6 ounces (170g) each
Elbows, cooked		2	Cup	Boil DRY elbows for 10 min in 4 qt pan; drain & set aside
Sausage,Hot Italian Homemade		8	Ounce	Break apart and fry; set aside
Butter		3	Tablespoon	Add to 8 cup glass bowl; melt in microwave; 1min
Flour, All Purpose		3	Tablespoon	wisk into melted butter
Pepper, Black ground		1/4	Teaspoon	add to bowl
Fennel seed		1/4	Teaspoon	Add to bowl; best if ground
****			CommentLine	grind and add to bowl
****			CommentLine	add to bowl and mix well with wisk
Milk; skim		1 1/2	Cup	add very slowly to bowl and wisk until smoothe
****			CommentLine	cook in microwave on hi until thick, wisk every minute
Cheese, Cheddar, brick		1	Pound	slice cheese thin and add to bowl
Cheese, Mozzarella,shreddeded, part skim		1/2	Cup	add to bowl; cook on high in microwave until cheese melts;
****			CommentLine	stir every minute
****			CommentLine	Add cooked sausage to bowl; stir
****			CommentLine	Add cooked elbows and stir
****			CommentLine	cook in microwave for 10 min; serve

Comments

Mac and cheese in not a very good choice for a kidney diet, so plan carefully

Serving Size(g) 170   About 6 oz.   Recipe Total Weight 1,412(g) About 49.8 oz.

Water	Calories	Protein	Fat	Carbs	Fiber	Sugars	Phos*	Pot*	Sodium*
100	413	22	29	16	1	3	402	228	496

*Values are in mg. All others are in grams

This is not a very kidney friendly recipe, but it can make a side dish if you plan for it and use small portions.

Meatballs, Italian

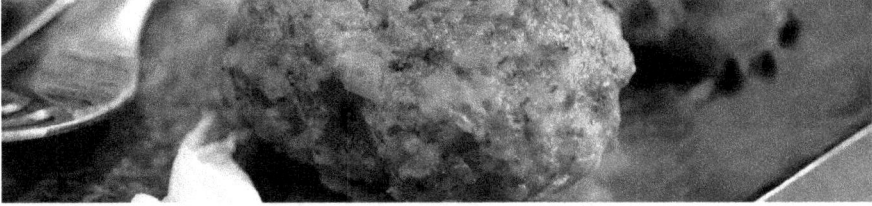

Item		Quantity	Directions
****		CommentLine	Makes about 34 meatballs which are about 35g cooked
Beef, Ground 80%; raw	2	Pound	Place into a large bowl
Bread Crumbs, dry	1 1/2	Cup	Add to bowl
Eggs, large	2	Each	Beat and Add to bowl
Cheese, Romano	1/2	Cup	Add to bowl
Parsley, dried	1/4	Cup	Add to bowl
Onion; medium; 110g	1/4	Cup	Chop and add to bowl
Oregano	1	Tablespoon	Add to bowl
Pepper, Black ground	1	Teaspoon	Add to bowl
Water, tap	1/2	Cup	Add to bowl, Mix
****		CommentLine	Place meatballs on greased cookie sheet
****		CommentLine	Bake in 400°F oven till 150°F; about 20 min
****		CommentLine	
****		CommentLine	Makes about

Comments

Use an ice cream scoop with a lever to release the molded meatballs. Push the meatball mix into the scoop to compact it and keep the meatball together

Serving Size(g) 140   About 4.9 oz.   Recipe Total Weight 1,454(g) About 51.3 oz.

Water	Calories	Protein	Fat	Carbs	Fiber	Sugars	Phos*	Pot*	Sodium*
61	345	22	22	13	1	1	271	321	346

*Values are in mg. All others are in grams

The meatballs are about the size of a golf ball and weigh about 25 grams or four fifths of an ounce.

Meatloaf

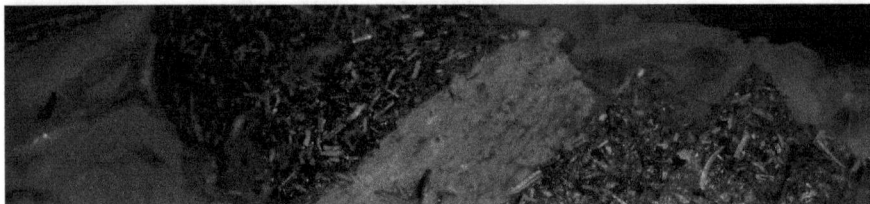

Item	Quantity		Directions
****	CommentLine		Makes 6 3/4 inch, 4 ounce (120g) slices
Beef, Ground 80%; raw	1	Pound	Add to large bowl
Cornmeal; yellow	1/2	Cup	add to bowl
Bread Crumbs, dry	1/2	Cup	Add to bowl
Ketchup	1/3	Cup	Add to bowl
Eggs, large	1	Each	add to bowl
Garlic, Granulated	1	Teaspoon	add to bowl
Basil, dried leaves	1	Teaspoon	add
Thyme, dried Leaves	1	Teaspoon	add to bowl
Parsley, dried	1	Teaspoon	add to bowl
Water, tap	1/2	Cup	Add to bowl & mix; place in 8.5 x 4.5 x 2.5 glass loaf pan. Cover with plastic wrap
****	CommentLine		cook in microwave; Power level 4 until 160 degrees F; about 15-20 min
****	CommentLine		See recipe for Meatball Sauce

Comments

Serve with meatloaf sauce--- This is good with a SMALL baked potato also with meatloaf sauce.

Serving Size(g) 120   About 4.2 oz.   Recipe Total Weight 831(g) About 29.3 oz.

Water	Calories	Protein	Fat	Carbs	Fiber	Sugars	Phos*	Pot*	Sodium*
73	255	14	15	16	1	3	158	274	234

*Values are in mg. All others are in grams

Meatloaf Sauce

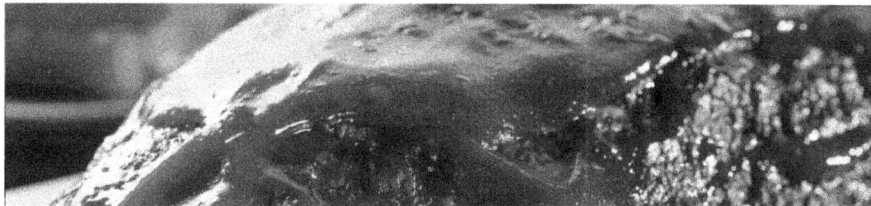

Item	Quantity		Directions
****		CommentLine	Makes about 6 servings, about 2 tablespoons each
Ketchup	1/2	Cup	Add to small bowl
Worcestershire Sauce	2	Tablespoon	add to bowl
Thyme, dried Leaves	1/4	Teaspoon	add to bowl
Oregano	1/4	Teaspoon	add to bowl
Pepper, Red ground	1/8	Teaspoon	Add to bowl, mix
****		CommentLine	Serving; 15 gm or ~.5oz per tbl; ~5gm per tsp

Comments

30 grams is about 2 tablespoons. ---Watch out, this sauce is a little high in sodium.

Serving Size(g) 30   About 1.1 oz.   Recipe Total Weight 171(g) About 6 oz.

Water	Calories	Protein	Fat	Carbs	Fiber	Sugars	Phos*	Pot*	Sodium*
21	29	0	0	8	0	6	10	117	295

*Values are in mg. All others are in grams

Omelet with Pepperoni

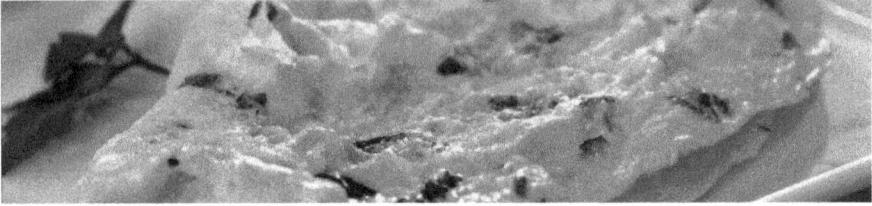

Item	Quantity		Directions
****		CommentLine	Makes 2 servings of 4.3 ounces (122g) each.
Eggs, large	3	Each	Whisk in bowl
Cream, heavy whipping	1	Tablespoon	Add to bowl and whisk
Pepper, Black ground	1/8	Teaspoon	Add to bowl and whisk
Garlic, Granulated	1/8	Teaspoon	Add to bowl and whisk
Onions, raw, tbsp chopped	2	Tablespoon	Dice Onion, set aside
Pepperoni, Sliced	6	Each	Dice, set aside
Cheese, Cheddar shredded	1/4	Cup	set aside
Butter, salted, pat (1" sq, 1/3" high)	1	Each	Add a pat of butter to fry pan
****		CommentLine	Melt butter in fry pan over medium low heat. When butter melts, pour egg mixture into pan.
****		CommentLine	Evenly distribute onion, pepperoni, cheddar cheese, and half the mozzarella cheese over the egg
Cheese, Mozzarella,shreddeded, part skim	1/8	Cup	When egg becomes firm, fold over in half, spread mozzarella cheese on top
****		CommentLine	Cook until cheese is melted, serve while hot.
****		CommentLine	

Comments
You can use garlic powder instead of granulated garlic, but not garlic salt. --

Serving Size(g) 122   About 4.3 oz.   Recipe Total Weight 245(g) About 8.6 oz.

Water	Calories	Protein	Fat	Carbs	Fiber	Sugars	Phos*	Pot*	Sodium*
81	263	16	21	3	0	1	269	170	358

Values are in mg. All others are in grams

Pork Pot Roast

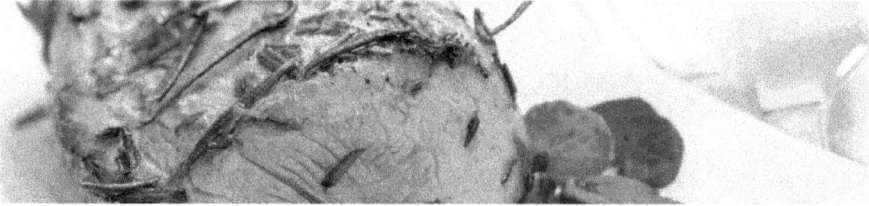

Item		Quantity	Directions
****		CommentLine	Serves 4
Pork, Shoulder, boston butt raw	2	Pound	Add to large fry pan with a tight lid
Pepper, Black ground	1/2	Teaspoon	Add to fry pan
Garlic, Granulated	1/2	Teaspoon	Add to pan
Sage, dry ground	1/2	Teaspoon	Add to fry pan
Marjoram, dried	1	Teaspoon	Add to pan
Water, tap	1	Cup	Add to fry pan; bring to boil; simmer 2 hrs;
****		CommentLine	Add water as necessary; bottom of pan should always be covered
****		CommentLine	Remove pork from pan; place on a platter; set aside
****		CommentLine	

Comments

Serve with Pot Roast Gravy --- See Gravy, Pot Roast

Serving Size(g) 120   About 4.2 oz.   Recipe Total Weight 1,145(g) About 40.4 oz.

Water	Calories	Protein	Fat	Carbs	Fiber	Sugars	Phos*	Pot*	Sodium*
90	178	17	12	0	0	0	182	307	59

* Values are in mg. All others are in grams

+

Pork Pot Roast Gravy

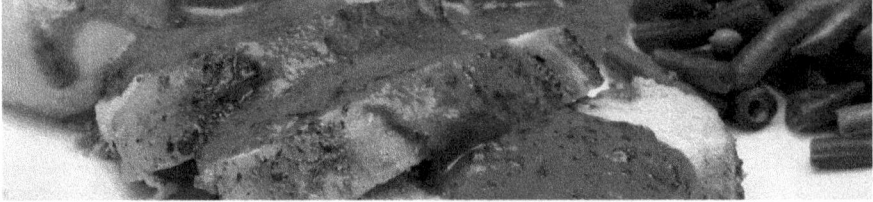

Item	Quantity		Directions
****	CommentLine		Makes about 4 cups of gravy
Soup, stock, beef, home-prepared, cup	1	Cup	Put meat on a platter. Pour liquid from pot roast pan into 4 cup Pyrex measure
Water, tap	2	Cup	Add water to make 3 cups; stir and return to fry pan on low heat
Flour, All Purpose	4	Tablespoon	Add flour to pint shaker jar with lid
Water, tap	1	Cup	Add water to flour in shaker jar; replace lid shake until all flour is mixed
****	CommentLine		Whisk flour mixture into fry pan; mix well
Sage, dry ground	1/2	Teaspoon	Add to fry pan;
Marjoram, dried	1/2	Teaspoon	Add to fry pan; mix well
****	CommentLine		Cook on medium heat; Stir constantly with spatula until thick; simmer for 2 more min. Serve
****	CommentLine		Add water if too thick. Add flour water mixture if too thin
****	CommentLine		

Comments

1/4 cup (4 tablespoons) of gravy is about 60 grams (2 oz) --A dash of salt is 155 milligrams of sodium -- so be careful if you add salt

Serving Size(g) 120   About 4.2 oz.   Recipe Total Weight 973(g) About 34.3 oz.

Water	Calories	Protein	Fat	Carbs	Fiber	Sugars	Phos*	Pot*	Sodium*
115	18	1	0	3	0	0	13	60	62

*Values are in mg. All others are in grams

Pork, General Toas

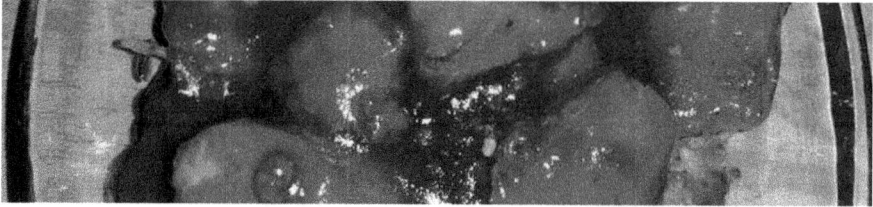

Item	Quantity		Directions
****		CommentLine	Serves 6
Pork, Shoulder, boston butt raw	1 1/2	Pound	Cut into 1/2 x 1 inch pieces; add to crock pot
Ginger, Ground	1	Teaspoon	Add to pot
Garlic, Minced	1	Teaspoon	Add to pot
Sugar, White	1/4	Cup	Add to pot
Pepper, Red ground	1/8	Teaspoon	Add to pot
Soy sauce, tamari		Tablespoon	Add to pot
Vinegar, Cider	1/2	Cup	Add to pot
Wine, table red	1/2	Cup	Add to pot
****		CommentLine	Cook in crock pot on low for 4 hours;

Comments

serve with rice or egg noodles

Serving Size(g) 120   About 4.2 oz.   Recipe Total Weight 974(g) About 34.4 oz.

Water	Calories	Protein	Fat	Carbs	Fiber	Sugars	Phos*	Pot*	Sodium*
84	198	15	10	7	0	6	166	304	53

*Values are in mg. All others are in grams

Pork, General Toas Stir Fry

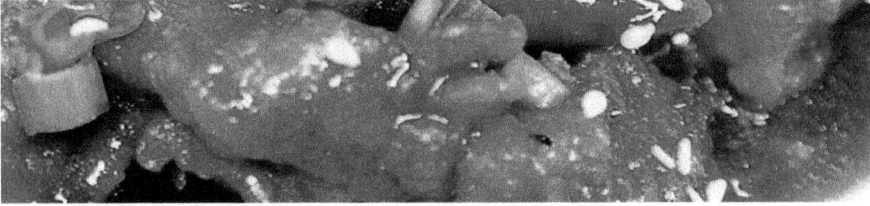

Item	Quantity		Directions
****	1	CommentLine	Makes about 4 servings,
****		CommentLine	Prepare the recipe for Gen Toas Sauce; set aside
Pork, Shoulder, boston butt raw	1	Pound	Slice pork 1/4 thick; then cut into 1 inch squares; set aside
Onion; medium; 110g	1	Each	Slice onion 1/4 inch thick; cut in half; set aside
Peppers, Bell, raw chopped	1/2	Each	Slice half a pepper into 1/4 inch strips; cut in half; set aside
Celery, raw, cup chopped	1	Cup	chop celery into 1/4 inch pieces, then cut in half; set aside
Vegetables, frozen, mixed	5	Ounce	Thaw 1/2 package of brocolli or oriental veggies; set aside
****		CommentLine	
Oil, Canola	2	Tablespoon	Add to large (12inch) pry pan; Place on medium heat
****		CommentLine	Add pork to pan; saute on medium heat until cooked;
Gen Toas Sauce	1	Cup	add Gen Toas Sauce to fry pan
****		CommentLine	Add onions, peppers, celery and veggies to fry pan; sauté for 5 minutes until veggies are tender
****	1	CommentLine	Add water if needed
****		CommentLine	

Comments

Serve over rice

Serving Size(g) 227   About 8 oz.   Recipe Total Weight 1,051(g) About 37.1 oz.

Water	Calories	Protein	Fat	Carbs	Fiber	Sugars	Phos'	Pot'	Sodium'
172	309	19	18	15	2	8	224	495	274

Values are in mg. All others are in grams

General Toas Sauce

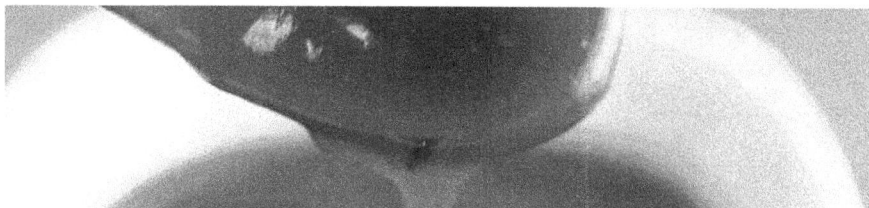

Item	Quantity		Directions
****		CommentLine	makes 14 ounces: almost 2 cups
Cornstarch	1 1/2	Tablespoon	Add to 2 cup glass measure
Ginger, Ground	2	Teaspoon	Add to 2 cup glass measure
Garlic, Minced	1/2	Teaspoon	Add to 2 cup glass measure
Sugar, White	1/4	Cup	Add to 2 cup glass measure
Pepper, Red ground	1/4	Teaspoon	Add to 2 cup glass measure, mix and set aside
Bouillon, Chicken, cube	1	Each	Place in 1 cup glass measure
Water, tap	1	Cup	add to 1 cup measure
****		CommentLine	Bring to boil in microwave; about 3 min. Stir till dissolved
Vinegar, Cider	2	Teaspoon	Add to 1 cup measure
Soy Sauce, shoyu, low sodium	1	Tablespoon	add to 1 cup measure
Wine, table red	1/4	Cup	add to 1 cup measure and stir
****		CommentLine	Slowly add to dry ingredients while stiring; mix well
****		CommentLine	cook in microwave until thick; about 4 minutes; stir every minute

Comments

No Comments have been entered.

Serving Size(g) 390   About 13.8 oz.   Recipe Total Weight 390(g) About 13.7 oz.

Water	Calories	Protein	Fat	Carbs	Fiber	Sugars	Phos*	Pot*	Sodium*
307	331	3	1	68	1	52	61	223	1,512

Values are in mg. All others are in grams

Gen Toas sauce is our version Gen Tso sauce. If you use it as a condiment, you will probably only use about two tablespoons (30gm).

Red Cabbage, Prepared

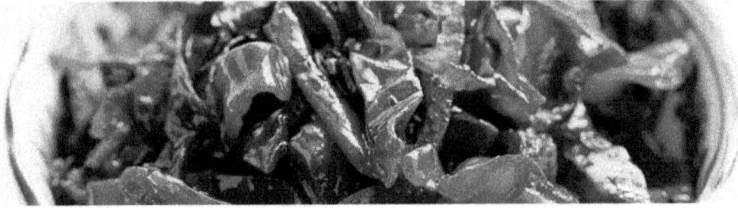

Item	Quantity		Directions
****		CommentLine	Makes a big pot full; about 9 servings, 4 ounces (120g) each
Cabbage, Red, Raw, shredded	8	Cup	Add 8 cups of shredded cabbage to 8 cup Pyrex measuring dish or bowl
Sugar, Brown	1/2	Cup	Add to dish
Vinegar, Cider	1/2	Cup	Add to dish
Water, tap	1	Cup	Add to dish
Bacon,thin slice, Uncooked	4	Each	Chop 4 slices into small pieces & add to dish
****		CommentLine	cook on power level 10 in micro wave; 40 min; or until tender; stir every 10 min
****		CommentLine	Check liquid in pot every 10 minutes; don't let the pot get dry

Comments

About 9 servings

Serving Size(g) 120   About 4.2 oz.   Recipe Total Weight 1,098(g) About 38.7 oz.

Water	Calories	Protein	Fat	Carbs	Fiber	Sugars	Phos*	Pot*	Sodium*
99	100	3	5	12	1	10	40	193	112

Values are in mg. All others are in grams

ried Rice

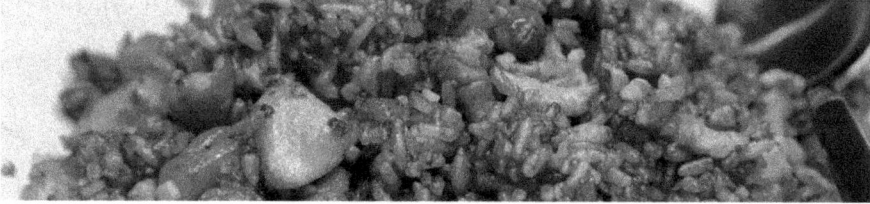

Item	Quantity		Directions
****		CommentLine	Makes about 7 servings, 8 ounces (277g) each
Rice, white long grain cooked	1	Cup	Add to 2 quart sauce pan
Water, tap	2	Cup	Add to pan and cover; bring to boil
****		CommentLine	Simmer on low heat for 14 minutes or until water is gone; set aside
Sausage;Hot Italian Homemade	12	Ounce	Add to large fry pan; cook and crumble
Ham, roasted, pork, cured, boneless, extra lean and regular	6	Ounce	dice and add to fry pan
Onion; medium; 110g	8	Tablespoon	Dice and add to pan
Mushrooms, white, raw	4	Ounce	Slice 6 medium mushrooms, add to pan
Garlic; Granulated	1	Teaspoon	Add to pan
Pepper; Black ground	1/4	Teaspoon	Add to pan;
Corn, frozen	1	Cup	Add to pan
Peas, Frozen	1	Cup	Add to pan
Water, tap	1/4	Cup	Add to pan
Soy Sauce, shoyu, low sodium	2	Teaspoon	add to pan;stir; simmer
Eggs, large	1	Each	Beat egg and add to pan; stir
****		CommentLine	Simmer until vegies are tender
****		CommentLine	Add cooked rice and cook on low heat for 5 min. serve

Comments

No Comments have been entered.

Serving Size(g) 227   About 8 oz.   Recipe Total Weight 1,727(g) About 60.9 oz.

Water	Calories	Protein	Fat	Carbs	Fiber	Sugars	Phos	Pot	Sodium
182	223	16	11	15	2	2	211	389	459

Values are in mg. All others are in grams

You need to plan ahead when eating fried rice. It is high in sodium and is nearly 25% of my daily sodium budget.

Rubin Sandwich with Red Cabbage

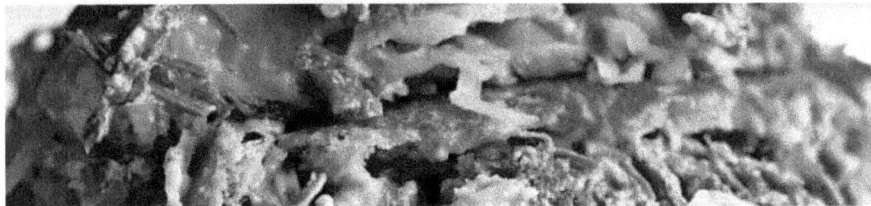

Item		Quantity	Directions
••••		CommentLine	Recipe is for 1 open face Rubin Sandwich
••••		CommentLine	Make Russian dressing ahead of time; set aside
••••		CommentLine	Warm 3 ounces (90 gm) of corned beef for each sandwich; set aside
••••		CommentLine	Warm 1/2 cup red cabbage for each sandwich in micro wave; set aside
Bread, Pumpernickel, 1oz slice	1	Each	
Butter, salted, pat (1" sq. 1/3" high)	1	Each	Spread small amount of butter on one side of bread
••••		CommentLine	Fry bread in a large fry pan or grill until bottom is toasted
Corned Beef	3	Ounce	Arrange evenly on toasted bread
Dressing, Russian	2	Tablespoon	Arrange evenly on corned beef
Red Cabbage, Cooked		Cup	Arrange evenly on sandwich
Cheese, Swiss slice	2	Each	Place Swiss cheese on top of cabbage
••••		CommentLine	Place sandwich in broiler until cheese is melted
••••		CommentLine	Serve while hot

Comments

Serve with extra Russian dressing

Serving Size(g) 186   About 6.6 oz.   Recipe Total Weight 186(g) About 6.6 oz.

Water	Calories	Protein	Fat	Carbs	Fiber	Sugars	Phos*	Pot*	Sodium*
88	525	28	36	21	2	5	395	373	1,329

Values are in mg. All others are in grams

Look at the sodium. This is a really bad choice even if you only eat half a sandwich which would give you a decent amount of protein. So, if you are going to eat a Red Rubin, plan ahead.

This is an example of how easy it is to break your budget.

Salsa, Homemade from Cans

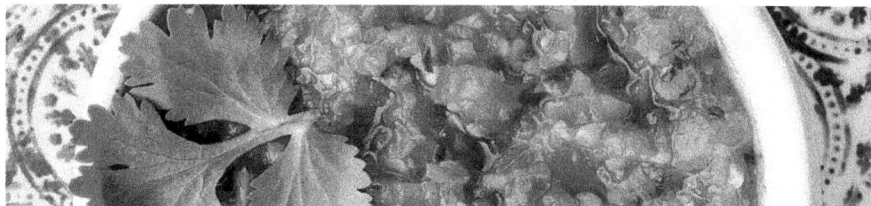

Item	Quantity		Directions
****		CommentLine	Makes about 15 servings; 2 tablespoons each; 1 ounce (30g)
Tomatoes, diced; can 15oz	1	Can	chop or coarsely grind 1 can of tomatoes add to 1 qt glass bowl
Peppers, Jalapeno canned	1	Ounce	Finely chop 1 oz of peppers, add to bowl
Onion; medium; 110g	1	Ounce	Chop 1 oz onion, add to bowl
Garlic, Granulated	1/4	Teaspoon	add garlic to bowl
Vinegar, Cider	2	Tablespoon	add vinegar to bowl
Sugar, White	1/4	Teaspoon	add sugar to bowl
Cilantro,(coriander) dried leaf	1/8	Teaspoon	add cilantro to bowl, mix
****		CommentLine	Simmer 5 minutes in microwave on PL10
****		CommentLine	Cool and serve

Comments

Serving size is 2 tablespoons or about 30 grams. 1 ounce. Number of servings is about 15

Serving Size(g) 30   About 1.1 oz.   Recipe Total Weight 515(g) About 18.1 oz.

Water	Calories	Protein	Fat	Carbs	Fiber	Sugars	Phos*	Pot*	Sodium*
27	10	0	0	2	1	1	9	80	74

*Values are in mg. All others are in grams

Sauce, Spaghetti Sauce with Meat

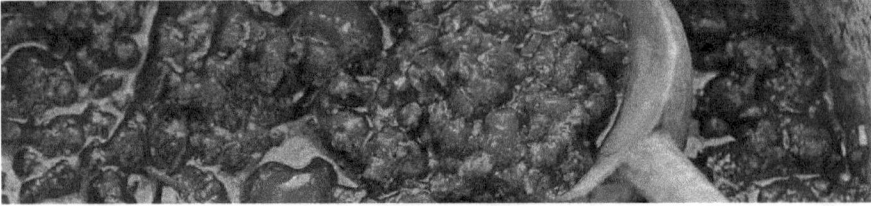

Item	Quantity		Directions
****		CommentLine	Makes about 3.5 quarts; shows 1/2 cup serving
Tomatos, Puree, 28oz can, no salt	3	Can	Add to large crock pot
Water, tap	1	Cup	add 1/2 can to pot
Oregano	1	Tablespoon	add to pot
Basil, dried leaves	1	Tablespoon	add to pot
Parsley, dried	1	Tablespoon	add to pot
Garlic, Minced	1	Tablespoon	add to pot
Sugar, White	2	Tablespoon	add to pot
Beef, Ground 80%; raw	8	Ounce	Crumble and add to pot
Sausage,Hot Italian Homemade	8	Ounce	crumble and add to pot
Pepper, Red ground	1/8	Teaspoon	add to pot; Cook in microwave on Hi until bubbling; about 25 min
****		CommentLine	Cook in crock pot on Hi for 4 hours
****		CommentLine	

Comments

Very high in potassium, so use sparingly.

Serving Size(g) 120   About 4.2 oz.   Recipe Total Weight 3,198(g) About 112.8 oz.

Water	Calories	Protein	Fat	Carbs	Fiber	Sugars	Phos*	Pot*	Sodium*
101	83	5	3	10	2	5	68	467	45

Values are in mg. All others are in grams

Sausage, Breakfast Homemade, Low Salt

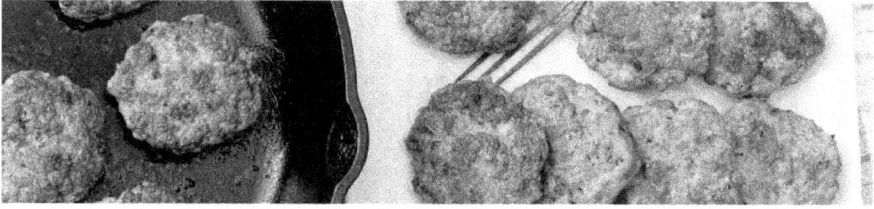

Item		Quantity	Directions
****		CommentLine	Makes 1 pound of sausage
Pork, Ground shoulder	1	Pound	Add ground pork to a medium size bowl, flatten out
Sausage seasoning , Breakfast Homemade; LOW salt	4	Teaspoon	Sprinkle 2 teaspoons of seasoning on meat. Fold over and press down
****		CommentLine	Sprinkle 2 teaspoons of seasoning on meat. Fold over and press down
****		CommentLine	Mix well using a big spoon. Keep folding over and mixing until evenly mixed

Comments

Much lower salt than bought breakfast sausage — Make 1 ounce patties and press thin. – Makes a good egg and sausage sandwich

Serving Size(g) 30   About 1.1 oz.   Recipe Total Weight 460(g) About 16.2 oz.

Water	Calories	Protein	Fat	Carbs	Fiber	Sugars	Phos	Pot	Sodium
19	71	5	5	0	0	0	54	93	78

Values are in mg. All others are in grams

Sausage, Breakfast Sausage Seasoning, Low Salt

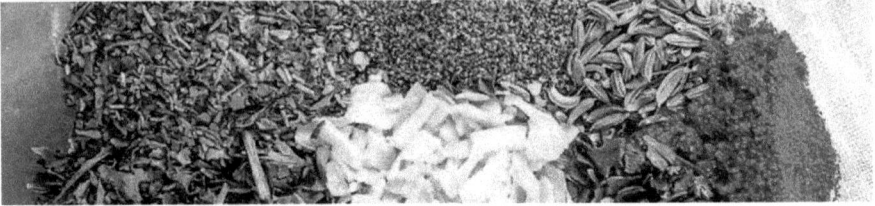

Item	Quantity		Directions
****		CommentLine	Makes enough for 3 pounds of pork. This is a Lower salt recipe
Sage, dry ground	2	Tablespoon	Add to small bowl
Marjoram, dried	1/2	Tablespoon	Add to bowl
Salt, table	1	Teaspoon	Add to bowl
Pepper, Black ground	1	Tablespoon	Add to bowl
****		CommentLine	Add to bowl, mix well, store in air tight jar
****		CommentLine	Use 4 teaspoons of mix for each pound of ground pork

Comments

No Comments have been entered

Serving Size(g) 19   About 0.7 oz.   Recipe Total Weight 19(g) About 0.7 oz.

Water	Calories	Protein	Fat	Carbs	Fiber	Sugars	Phos*	Pot*	Sodium*
1	33	1	1	8	4	0	16	152	2.669

*Values are in mg. All others are in grams

Sausage, Hot Italian Homemade

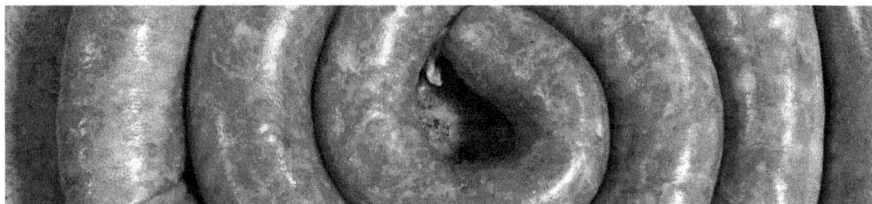

Item	Quantity		Directions
****		CommentLine	Makes about 8 servings, 4 ounces (113g) each
Pork, Ground shoulder	2	Pound	Add ground pork to medium bowl; flatten out
Italian Sausage Seasoning	1 1/2	Tablespoon	Spread evenly on pork; Fold over and mix until evenly mixed

Comments

Yummy --- a big Kitchen Ade mixer is real handy for doing this.

Serving Size(g) 113   About 4 oz.   Recipe Total Weight 917(g) About 32.4 oz.

Water	Calories	Protein	Fat	Carbs	Fiber	Sugars	Phos*	Pot*	Sodium*
72	267	19	20	0	0	0	206	353	184

*Values are in mg. All others are in grams

Sausage Seasoning, Hot Italian

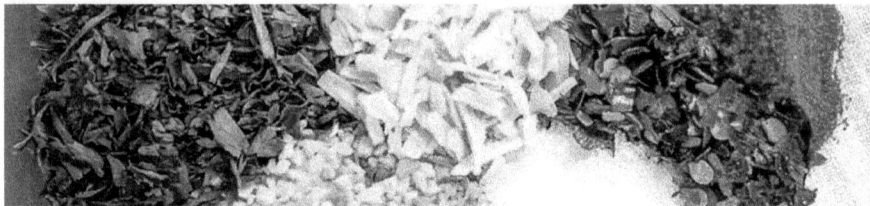

Item	Quantity		Directions
~~		CommentLine	Makes 16 pounds of medium hot sausage
Pepper, Red ground	2	Tablespoon	Add to small bowl
Pepper, Crushed red	2	Tablespoon	Add to bowl
Pepper, Black ground	2	Tablespoon	Add to bowl
Fennel seed	1/4	Cup	Add to bowl
Basil, dried leaves	2	Tablespoon	Add to bowl
Salt, table	1	Tablespoon	Add to bowl and mix well
~~		CommentLine	use 3/4 Tbl of mix per pound of ground pork for medium hot

Comments

Enough to make 16 pounds of Kidney friendly Italian Sausage ---3/4 table spoon is a serving size of 4 8 grams; --this makes 1 pound of medium hot sausage

Serving Size(g) 5   About 0.2 oz.   Recipe Total Weight 83(g) About 2.9 oz.

Water	Calories	Protein	Fat	Carbs	Fiber	Sugars	Phos*	Pot*	Sodium*
0	11	0	0	2	1	0	12	65	458

*Values are in mg. All others are in grams

Scrapple

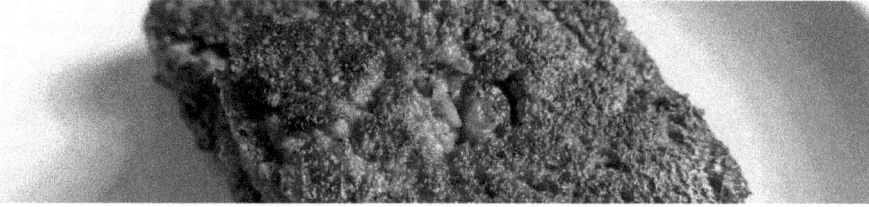

Item	Quantity		Directions
****		CommentLine	Makes 2 loaf pans 8.5x4.5x2.5
Pork, Shoulder, boston butt raw	2	Pound	Cut to 1 inch thick strips, add to 4 qt pot
Water, tap	4	Cup	Add water to pot to cover meat
Sage, dry ground	1	Tablespoon	Add to pot
Pepper, Black ground	2	Teaspoon	Add to pot
Salt, table	1/2	Teaspoon	Add to pot
Thyme, dried Leaves	2	Teaspoon	Add to pot
Savory, ground	2	Teaspoon	Add to pot
****		CommentLine	Simmer Pork until shredable; about 2 hrs
****		CommentLine	pour stock into 8 cup measure cup
Water, tap	2	Cup	Add water to stock to make 4 cups
****		CommentLine	Shred the pork, return to pot
****		CommentLine	Return stock to pot & bring to boil
Cornmeal, yellow	2	Cup	Place in 4 cup measure cup
Water, tap	1 1/2	Cup	Add to corn meal, stir
****		CommentLine	Remove stock from heat; Slowly add corn meal to stock; Stir constantly
****		CommentLine	Stir & cook mixture until very thick; at least 3 minutes; Stir constantly
****		CommentLine	Press tightly into 2 loaf pans; cool and let set.
****		CommentLine	Cut into 3/8 inch slices. Fry over med heat until crisp.
****		CommentLine	

Comments

Good with eggs and toast,---made with pork only; no scraps or organ meat

Serving Size(g) 120   About 4.2 oz.   Recipe Total Weight 2,917(g) About 102.9 oz.

Water	Calories	Protein	Fat	Carbs	Fiber	Sugars	Phos*	Pot*	Sodium*
99	107	7	5	8	1	0	96	152	83

*Values are in mg. All others are in grams

Soup, Lentil

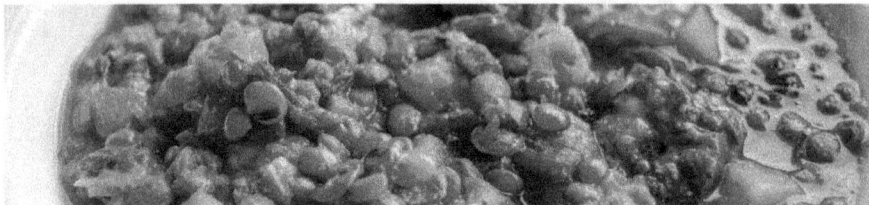

Item	Quantity		Directions
****		CommentLine	Makes about 6 servings; 8 ounces (227g) each
Lentils, Dry	1/2	Pound	Add to 4 Qt pot
Water, tap	4	Cup	Add to 4 Qt pot
Ham, unheated, pork, cured, boneless, extra lean and regular	1/2	Cup	Diced, Add to pot
Sausage, Hot Italian Homemade	1/4	Pound	Crumble & add to pot
Marjoram, dried	1/2	Teaspoon	Add to pot
Oregano	1/4	Teaspoon	Add to pot
Pepper, Black ground	1/2	Teaspoon	Add to pot
Onions, raw, cup, chopped	1/2	Cup	Dice onion, add to pot
****		CommentLine	Bring to boil then simmer on low heat until lentils are soft, about 20 min

Comments

No Comments have been entered.

Serving Size(g) 227   About 8 oz.   Recipe Total Weight 1,427(g) About 50.3 oz.

Water	Calories	Protein	Fat	Carbs	Fiber	Sugars	Phos`	Pot`	Sodium`
182	194	14	5	25	4	1	165	357	179

Values are in mg. All others are in grams

Taco Meat

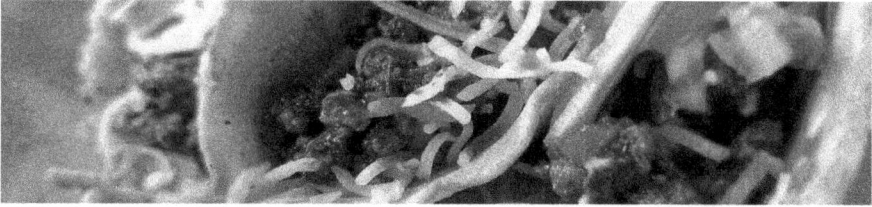

Item	Quantity		Directions
****		CommentLine	Makes about 6 servings, 4 ounces (115g) each
Beef, Ground 80%; raw	1	Pound	Add to large fry pan; cook & remove melted fat
Garlic, Granulated	1	Teaspoon	Add to pan
Ketchup	3/4	Cup	Add 3/4 cup to pan
Hot Sauce, Franks	2	Tablespoon	Add to pan
Pepper, Red ground	1/4	Teaspoon	Add to pan
Chili Powder, Homemade	1	Teaspoon	Add to pan; simmer for 5 min

Comments

Easy, quick recipe for making tacos

Serving Size(g) 115   About 4.1 oz.   Recipe Total Weight 694(g) About 24.5 oz.

Water	Calories	Protein	Fat	Carbs	Fiber	Sugars	Phos*	Pot*	Sodium*
74	229	13	15	10	0	7	132	339	358

*Values are in mg. All others are in grams

Teriyaki Sauce

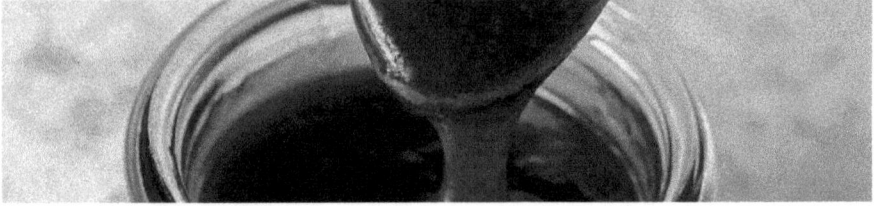

Item	Quantity		Directions
****		CommentLine	Makes about 5 cups; serving size is 2 tablespoons
Cornstarch	1 1/2	Teaspoon	Add to 2 cup glass measuring cup
Ginger, Ground	2	Teaspoon	Add to glass cup
Garlic, Granulated	1/2	Teaspoon	Add to glass cup
Sugar, White	1/4	Cup	Add to glass cup; mix and set aside
Bouillon, Chicken, cube	1	Each	Add to 1cup glass measuring cup
Water, tap	1	Cup	Add to 1cup glass measuring cup
****		CommentLine	Bring to a boil in microwave, about 3 minutes. Stir until dissolved
Vinegar, Cider	2	Teaspoon	Add to 1cup glass measuring cup
Wine, table red	1/4	Cup	Add to 1cup glass measuring cup; Stir
****		CommentLine	Slowly add to dry ingredients while stirring; mix well
****		CommentLine	cook in microwave on high until thick, about 4 minutes; stir every minute
****	1	CommentLine	serve warm

Comments

No Comments have been entered.

Serving Size(g) 30   About 1.1 oz.   Recipe Total Weight 366(g) About 12.9 oz.

Water	Calories	Protein	Fat	Carbs	Fiber	Sugars	Phos*	Pot*	Sodium*
24	24	0	0	5	0	4	3	13	79

*Values are in mg. All others are in grams

Tuna and Noodles

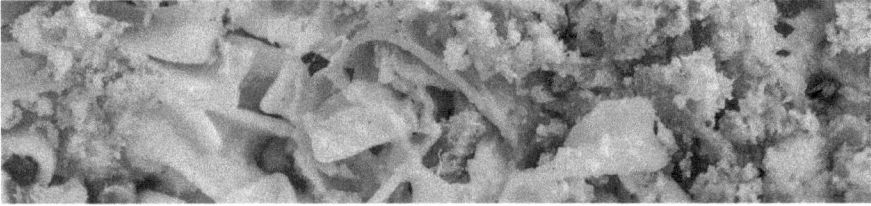

Item	Quantity		Directions
****		CommentLine	Makes 10 servings; 4 ounces (115g) each
Noodles, egg cooked	8	Ounce	Boil 8 oz noodles in 8cup pot for 10 minutes; drain and set aside
Tunafish in water (5 oz can)	3	Can	Add to large glass dish
Soup, Cream of Mushroom	1	Can	Add to large glass dish
Pepper, Black ground	1	Teaspoon	Add to glass dish
Milk; skim	1/2	Cup	Add to large glass dish
****		CommentLine	Add cooked noodles to glass dish, mix
Cheese, American Sliced	6	Each	Layer cheese in middle and top of noodles
****	5	CommentLine	Cook in microwave on power level 7 until cheese is melted
****		CommentLine	stir every minute after cheese starts to melt

Comments

This is not a kidney friendly recipe, --There is too much salt-- so be caaraeful how much you eat.

Serving Size(g) 115   About 4.1 oz.   Recipe Total Weight 1,249(g) About 44 oz.

Water	Calories	Protein	Fat	Carbs	Fiber	Sugars	Phos*	Pot*	Sodium*
85	146	12	7	9	0	1	187	138	556

*Values are in mg All others are in grams

This is another recipe that you need to plan ahead before eating. It is high in sodium and a little low in protein. So be careful.

Tuna, Creamed

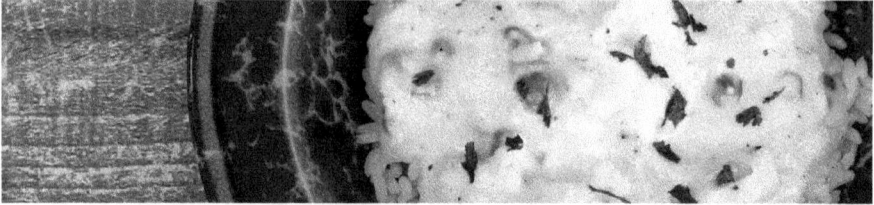

Item	Quantity		Directions
****	1	CommentLine	Makes about 8 servings; 4 ounces (115g) each
Butter	3	Tablespoon	Add to 1 quart pyrix dish; melt in micro wave about 1 minute
Flour, All Purpose	3	Tablespoon	Add to 1qt bowl
Salt, table	1/8	Teaspoon	Add to 1qt bowl; mix with wisk until smoothe
Milk; skim	1 1/2	Cup	Slowly add to bowl while wisking briskly; mix well
****		CommentLine	Microwave on high stirring every minute until thick
Tunafish in water (5 oz can)	2	Can	Flake and Add to 1qt bowl
Poultry Seasoning, Homemade	1/2	Teaspoon	Add to 1qt bowl
Pepper, Black ground	1/8	Teaspoon	Add to 1qt bowl
Peas, Frozen	1/2	Cup	Add to 1qt bowl
Corn, frozen	1/2	Cup	Add to 1qt bowl; mix well
****		CommentLine	Cook in microwave for 5 minutes on high stirring every minute
****		CommentLine	Serve on toast or baking powder biscuits

Comments

Serve on toast or biscuits,--- careful of sodium

Serving Size(g) 115   About 4.1 oz.   Recipe Total Weight 857(g) About 30.2 oz.

Water	Calories	Protein	Fat	Carbs	Fiber	Sugars	Phos*	Pot*	Sodium*
90	120	10	5	9	1	3	124	191	206

*Values are in mg. All others are in grams

Chapter 7: Resources to Get More Info

KDC Food Finder: https://kidneyfoodfinder.com

Kidney Diet Central: https://KidneyDietCentral.com

Kidney Diet Central Facebook Page:
https://www.facebook.com/KidneyDietCentral

Dialysis Newbies Facebook Group:
https://KidneyDietCentral.com/newbies

USDA Food Data Central: https://fdc.nal.usda.gov

Kidney School: https://KidneySchool.org

Home Dialyzors United (HDU): https://HomeDialyzorsUnited.org

Facebook Group: https://kidneydietcentral.com/HDU-group

Home Dialysis Central: https://www.kidney.org

Facebook Group: https://kidneydietcentral.com/HomeDialysis

Help, I Need Dialysis:
https://kidneydietcentral.com/help-I-need-dialysis

National Kidney Foundation: https://www.kidney.org

American Kidney Fund: https://www.KidneyFund.org

Track your diet pdf spread sheet:
https://kidneydietcentral.com/spreadsheet-pdf

Track your diet Excel spread sheet:
https://kidneydietcentral.com/spreadsheet

Chapter 8: Weight & Measures Equivalent Chart

Quickly & Easily

Convert Standard Measures to Grams

or

Convert Grams to Standard Measure

Unit	Grams	Equals
Teaspoon	5	1 Teaspoon
Tablespoon	15	3 Teaspoons
1/4 Cup	60	4 Tablespoons
1/3 Cup	76	5 1/3 ounces
1/2 Cup	114	4 ounces
Cup	227	8 ounces
Pint	454	16 ounces
Ounce	30	2 Tablespoons
Pound	454	1 Pint

Chapter 9: Nutrient List

This chart is a quick reference showing the nutrient values of 100 grams of several different foods. 100 grams is about 3 to 4 ounces.

Food Name	Per 100 Grams				
	Protein	Phos.	Potas.	Sodium	Calories
Protein, Unjury, Unflavored	84	253	549	148	338
Protein, Unjury, Strawberry	78	241	352	204	370
Protein, Unjury Chocolate	78	259	556	315	370
Turkey, white, roasted	30	230	249	99	147
Beef, Sirloin	30	265	437	72	257
Peanut Butter, salted	25	358	649	459	588
Pork	25	208	305	58	267
Hamburg	24	194	270	59	286
pepperoni	23	200	300	1700	500
Shrimp, cooked	23	306	170	294	119
Chicken	21	210	320	116	114
Scallops, cooked	21	426	314	667	111
Talapia	20	247	350	27	89
ham	20	260	325	1269	122
Taco meat	18	152	295	248	233
Meatballs	17	164	214	112	225
Tuna Salad	16	137	291	365	124
Sausage	15	173	250	128	290
Macaroni Salad	14	180	251	808	507
Egg	13	198	138	142	143
pasta	13	162	197	2	369
bacon	12	188	208	833	458
scrapple	6	76	117	60	132

About the Authors

Bill

Bill is an electronic engineer with a degree from Syracuse University. He has been solving engineering problems for 55 years. The most difficult problem he faced was when Sue, his wife, was diagnosed with kidney failure and needed to start dialysis. Like everyone else needing to start dialysis, He and Sue had no idea of what or how much Sue could eat. He then developed a spreadsheet to track her daily nutrition. Every meal they would sit at the table with a scale and a laptop. They were very successful at maintaining her diet. In the eight years Sue was on a kidney diet, her labs were always within the required limits, and she felt good.

Susan

Susan Emeny, a career software engineer for over 30 years was diagnosed with kidney failure in March of 2012 and started dialysis July 26, 2012. After suffering through many infections and different types of dialysis, the right prescription was found in March of 2016. Through all this time, she and her husband have been monitoring her diet with software she began developing in the spring of 2012. On Sept. 22, 2019 she received a kidney transplant and is now doing well.